Treatment Protocols
for
Language Disorders in Children

Volume I
Essential Morphologic Skills

Treatment Protocols
for
Language Disorders in Children

Volume I
Essential Morphologic Skills

M. N. Hegde, Ph.D.

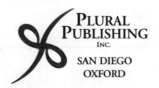

**PLURAL
PUBLISHING**
INC.

SAN DIEGO
OXFORD

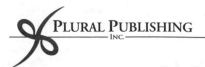

5521 Ruffin Road
San Diego, CA 92123

e-mail: info@pluralpublishing.com
Web site: http://www.pluralpublishing.com

49 Bath Street
Abington, Oxfordshire OX14 1EA
United Kingdom

Typeset in 10/12 Bookman by Flanagan's Publishing Services, Inc.
Printed in the United States of America by McNaughton and Gunn

ISBN-13: 978-1-59756-045-0
ISBN-10: 1-59756-045-6
Library of Congress Control Number: 2005908628

Contents

Preface

The *Webster's II New College Dictionary* defines a protocol as, "a plan for a scientific experiment or treatment." An effective plan for treatment needs to be as clear and precise as a scientific experiment. The concept of protocols, therefore, is eminently suitable for treatment plans in speech-language pathology.

Treatment in communication disorders is primarily a matter of planned social interaction. These interactions can be envisioned as dynamic relationships in which the clinician and the client affect each other. A single observation of a treatment session will convince us that, in any treatment session, the clinician and the client simply play out their respective roles and come out of successful treatment as changed persons. It is this view of treatment that has inspired these protocols.

If treatment is a set of scenarios in which the clinician and the client play out their roles, protocols are scripts they follow to achieve improved patterns of communication. Therefore, these protocols are written as scripts to help the clinician and the client play their roles effectively, efficiently, and with a reasonable expectation of positive outcome for the child and his or her family.

This is the first of two books on protocols for treating language disorders in children. This book includes protocols to establish basic language skills in most children with language disorders. The protocols concentrate on teaching morphologic skills. Deficient morphologic skills are diagnostic of language disorders in children. Therefore, teaching the production of morphologic skills is an essential part of speech-language pathologists' clinical work with children who have language disorders.

Protocols for teaching more advanced language skills are included in a second volume, *Treatment Protocols for Language Disorders in Children: Social Communication*. This volume includes protocols for teaching conversational skills and narrative skills. Together, it is hoped that the two volumes cover a comprehensive range of skills that speech-language pathologists find themselves teaching children with language disorders.

Introduction to Treatment Protocols and the CD Resource

These protocols for treating language disorders in children are written as scenarios that unfold in teaching morphologic skills to children. Clinicians who treat children with language disorders spend significant amounts of time and effort in establishing morphologic skills. Unless morphologic deficiencies, which characterize virtually all children with language disorders, are addressed, advanced language intervention is not possible. Therefore, this first in a series of two books on child language treatment concentrates on morphologic features. The second volume extends the protocols to social communication, including pragmatic language skills.

In selecting treatment procedures for the protocols, the overriding concern has been efficacy. The protocols, therefore, include a core set of treatment procedures for which there is plenty of replicated positive evidence.

Evidential Basis of the Treatment Protocols

Evidence-based treatment in speech-language pathology should be based on controlled scientific experiments that evaluate the effects of individual procedures. Treatment procedures that receive controlled experimental support may be recommended for general practice. If the evidence is widely replicated, the procedures may be somewhat standard and consistent across varied target behaviors. In preparing these protocols, evidence has been the most overriding concern. The main treatment procedures included in the protocols are well-researched behavioral techniques of modeling, prompting, fading, shaping, positive reinforcement, and corrective feedback (Hegde & Maul, 2006).

Although this is not meant to be a review of child language treatment research, a few historical trends may be recognized. The earliest treatment efficacy studies on teaching morphologic features to children with language disorders, conducted as early as the 1960s and 1970s and continued since then, showed that behavioral techniques and the discrete trial procedure to be effective (see, for example, Guess, 1969; Guess & Baer, 1973; Guess, et al., 1968; Hart, 1985; Hegde, 1980; Hegde & Gierut, 1979; Hegde & McConn, 1981; Hegde, Noll, & Pecora, 1979; Risley & Reynolds, 1970; Schumaker & Sherman, 1970, among others, for a sampling of early experimental studies). Over the years, the evidence for these techniques and procedures has been replicated by many studies. Research has included such diverse populations as children with specific language impairment, mental retardation, hearing impairment, autism, or other developmental disabilities. Furthermore, research also has documented the effectiveness of the procedures in teaching a variety of language skills. The American Speech-Language-Hearing Association's (ASHA) (2005) child language treatment efficacy data base on its Web site lists more than 170 studies on treatment efficacy; the majority of those studies have documented the usefulness of such commonly used techniques as modeling, prompting, shaping, positive reinforcement, and corrective feedback—all implemented within discrete trial formats. Clinicians may visit the ASHA Web site (www.asha.org/members/research/NOMS2child_language.htm) and consult various printed sources for bibliographies and review of behavioral research on child language treatment (see, for instance, Bricker, 1993; Goldstein, 2002; Hegde, 1998; Hegde & Maul, 2006; Kaiser & Gray, 1993; Koegel, Koegel, & Dunlap, 1996; Maurice, 1996;

Reichle & Wacker, 1993; Warren, 1992; Warren & Kaiser, 1986; Warren & Rogers Warren, 1985 for a review and summary of child language treatment research). Because they are based on replicated efficacy data across varied children and language targets, the protocols described in this book are relatively standard and consistent across child language treatment targets.

What the Protocols Offer

Treatment protocols are common in medicine, where such protocols are more prescriptive. Treatment plans in speech-language pathology need to be flexible and adaptable to individual clients. The protocols described in this book leave much room for the clinician's innovation, adaptation, and modification. The protocols for each language skill are described as a separate and complete entity. All target behaviors may be taught in a simple and predictable manner. For instance, protocols show that treating each target skill involves the following:

- **A protocol to establish baserates** of target skills in a child. The baserates help establish the need for treatment and provide an objective and quantitative basis to evaluate the child's progress in treatment.
- **A baserate recording sheet** that lists up to 20 exemplars of a language target along with columns for two types of baserate trials: a set of evoked trials and a set of modeled trials; the clinician may copy the page and use it in the clinic to obtain reliable baserates.
- **A protocol to teach the skill** that provides unfolding scenarios for treatment; the protocols are detailed enough for the clinician to implement treatment with little or no modifications; the protocols are written in the form of scripts for both the clinician and the child; in essence, these treatment protocols allow the clinician and the client to play their respective roles.
- **A treatment recording sheet** that lists up to 10 target exemplars that may be taught in discrete trials or more naturalistic interactions; the recording sheet provides for objective measurement of each attempt the child makes with and without modeling.
- **A protocol to probe for generalized production** of new exemplars with no training; these probe protocols, too, are written in the form of scripts that assign roles the clinician and the child play.
- **A probe recording sheet** to document the percent correct generalized response of the skill just taught; these probe protocols also help determine whether the child needs to be taught additional exemplars; if the child meets the probe criterion, the clinician then can move on to other target skill or to a higher level of training.

The protocols for most language skills, then, have five elements, each formatted on a single page: (1) the baserate protocol, (2) the baserate recording sheet, (3) the treatment protocol, (4) the treatment recording sheet, and (5) the probe protocol and probe recording sheet. For a few target skills that are sequenced from single words to phrases to sentences, probes may be skipped for early or intermediate skills. For instance, there is no need to probe for generalized production of a grammatic morpheme at the phrase level. Probes at the sentence production level are, of course, important. Therefore, protocols for some target behaviors are formatted on four pages (skipping the page for probe protocols and probe recording sheet).

Each clinician, however, may sequence the target skills in any number of ways to suit an individual child. The entry point for a child may be anywhere within the sequence. Clinicians may select any of the skills that are considered appropriate, functional, and useful to the child. In some cases, the sequence and the entry point may depend on certain prerequisite skills. For example, before teaching the auxiliary *is* or *was*, the clinician needs to teach a child the production of the present progressive *ing*.

Clinicians may use the recording sheets to document the child's progress in treatment. The clinician who uses these protocols may document the systematic changes in the child's skill level across the treatment sessions. Because they are objective and show positive changes from the baserate level of the skill, the data recorded will help document the child's improvement under treatment and should support any claims for third-party reimbursement for services.

In most cases, the clinician can simply photocopy a page from the printed book to use in the treatment sessions. For instance, the clinician can photocopy a baserate or treatment recording sheet that contains all the target exemplars already printed on it. This will save the treatment planning and preparation time as well as considerable effort involved in generating extensive exemplars (words, phrases, and sentences to be taught). The baserate, treatment, and probe recording sheets are also provided in Appendixes and can be photocopies by clinicians for personal use. Furthermore, the clinician can use the CD, as described next, to prepare for treatment sessions and to generate customized forms.

The book includes a glossary that is more detailed than the usual. All treatment terms are defined and described in some detail with examples. Clinicians who are unfamiliar with some of the terms used in the protocols are encouraged to review the detailed glossary.

How to Use the Accompanying CD

The CD that accompanies the book contains all the baserate, treatment, and probe recording sheets. All the files on the CD are modifiable. The clinician can type in new information or delete what is on them. This makes it possible for the clinician to individualize treatment for particular children. For instance, the clinician can easily delete an exemplar and type in one that is more specific to the child. In baserating, teaching, and probing functional words, the clinician can type in the names of family members, teachers, pets, friends, favorite food items, favorite activities, and so forth. While individualizing the recording sheets in this manner, the clinician can retain the standard recording sheet given on the CD.

To further individualize the recording sheets, the clinician can type in the name of the clinic or the school, the child's name, the clinician's name, date of treatment session, and such other clinician- and child-specific information that are typically included on recording sheets. Unlike the typical forms given in resource books, the modifiable and printable forms on the CD do not have page numbers, book chapter titles, and other information that would make the forms inappropriate to place in a client's folder. Forms printed (or even photocopied from the Appendix) will look like the clinician's clinic stationery.

For the clinician's convenience, the CDs are prepared in simple MS Word format, which most clinicians are familiar with; the CD is not encrypted in any way to facilitate quick access and easy use of the documents on it. Once again, use of the CD will help the clinician save planning time and effort involved in preparing for treatment sessions.

An Overview of Treatment Procedures and Sequence

The treatment procedures included in the protocols are systematic and well-sequenced. As noted in the Introduction, both the procedures and their sequence are supported by treatment efficacy research. Treatment for a given child is typically started after an assessment is made. The protocols assume that an assessment has been completed.

Distinguishing a Skill from an Exemplar

To understand the structure and sequence implied in the treatment protocols, it is essential to distinguish a target skill from an exemplar. For example, (1) production of the regular plural *s*, (2) adjectives, (3) passive sentences, or (4) *wh*-questions illustrate four distinct and independent **target skills**. Each target skill, however, is taught with multiple exemplars. An exemplar is one instance or an example of a target skill.

For example:

- "I see two cups," "these are five cats," and "I have nine books" are exemplars of the target skill regular plural *s*.
- "This is a big house," "That is a small ant," and "I see a blue book" are three exemplars of adjectives.
- "The ball was kicked by the boy" and "the cat was chased by the dog" are two exemplars of passive sentences.
- "What is this?" and "What is that?" are two exemplars of *wh*-questions.

It is only by teaching specific exemplars that a clinician establishes a target skill or behavior in a child. To master a skill, some children need to be taught more exemplars than others. The protocols include up to 20 exemplars for each target skill. All are baserated, some are taught, and those that are not taught are probed for generalized productions.

Establishing the Baserates

Following the assessment, the clinician's first job is to baserate the skills that will be taught in the initial treatment sessions. Baserates are in-depth assessments of selected target skills. Going beyond the traditional assessment, baserates help ensure that the child indeed needs treatment for the selected target skill. Because each target skill is baserated with some 20 or so exemplars (opportunities to produce the skill), the results of baserate procedures are more extensive, as well as more reliable, than the traditional assessment results. Baserates help assess the child's improvement during the treatment process. Even more importantly, baserates help justify positive outcomes for the child and thus support claims for reimbursement.

When treatment fails to produce significant improvement over the baserate levels, the clinician can modify the treatment procedure. For example, the clinician may select more effective reinforcers for the child, simplify the target skills, select another target skill, model more frequently, use the shaping procedure, and so forth. Without a reliable baserate, prompt treatment modifications are difficult to make because the clinician does not know whether the skills being treated are improving or not.

There are two kinds of baserate trials: modeled and evoked. On modeled trials, the clinician asks a question and immediately produces the correct response for the child to imitate. On evoked trials, the clinician does not model. Both kinds of trials are administered for each exemplar.

Each kind of baserate trial has a standard structure. On the modeled baserate trial, the clinician:

- presents a stimulus picture or object; for example, the clinician presents two books or a picture of two books
- points to the stimulus and asks a question; for example, "Johnny, what do you see? [what are these?]"
- immediately after asking the question, the clinician models the correct response; for example, the clinician says, "Johnny, say, two books," and waits for a few seconds for the child to respond
- the clinician scores the child's response as correct, incorrect, or absent (no response); then waits for a few seconds to initiate the next trial
- the clinician then introduces the next trial; presents a different picture (e.g., two cups), asks the question, models the response, scores the child's response, and moves on to the next exemplar

On evoked baserate trial, the clinician simply skips modeling. After presenting the stimulus, asks a question, waits for the child to respond, and scores the response.

An important aspect of baserates is that the child receives no differential feedback (reinforcement or corrective feedback) for correct or incorrect responses. Absence of such feedback distinguishes a baserate trial from a treatment trial.

Implementing Treatment

After establishing the baserates, the clinician initiates treatment. As the protocols make clear, the baserate and treatment trials have a similar structure. The treatment trials include all steps of baserate trials; in addition, they include verbal praise or corrective feedback.

Treatment trials begin with modeling. Eventually, modeling is faded to introduce the evoked trials. On a modeled treatment trial, the clinician:

- presents a stimulus picture or object; for example, the clinician presents two books or a picture of two books
- points to the stimulus and asks a question; for example, "Johnny, what do you see? [what are these?]"
- immediately after asking the question, the clinician models the correct response; for example, the clinician says, "Johnny, say, two book**s**," vocally emphasizing the target morpheme, and waits for a few seconds for the child to respond
- reinforces the child's correct responses (e.g., "Excellent!" or "That was correct!") or offers corrective feedback (e.g., "No, that was not correct! You should have said . . . ")
- the clinician then scores the child's response as correct, incorrect, or absent (no response) and waits for a few seconds to initiate the next trial

- the clinician then introduces the next trial; presents a different picture (e.g., two cups), asks the question, models the response, offers appropriate feedback, scores the child's response, and moves on to the next exemplar

When the child gives 5 correctly imitated responses in a sequence, the clinician fades modeling to introduce the evoked trials. Responses are *evoked* when there is no modeling and *imitated* when there is modeling. Two standard methods of fading modeling into an evoked trial is to use the partial modeling (Say, these are two . . . ") and hinting ("Did you forget something?" or "Don't forget the *s* at the end of the word *book.*")

An important aspect of treatment trials is the prompt reinforcement or corrective feedback given to the child. Again, this is what distinguishes a treatment trial from a baserate trial.

Sequencing Treatment

Several clinical criteria help move the child in a smooth and efficient manner through the various stages of treatment. Essentially, the clinician should judge when to discontinue modeling on a given exemplar, when to stop teaching a given exemplar, when to probe for generalized productions, and when to move on to the next level of training involving the same target skill or when to move on to the next (different) target skill. The following clinical criteria help make those judgments:

- **When to discontinue modeling.** When the child gives five consecutively correct, imitated responses on a given exemplar, fade modeling with partial modeling or hints.
- **When to reintroduce modeling.** When the child makes errors on the first few evoked trials, reintroduce modeling and fade it again after about five correct, imitated responses.
- **When to stop teaching an exemplar.** When the child gives 10 consecutively correct, evoked responses on a given exemplar (e.g., saying "two books" on 10 consecutive evoked trials while teaching the regular plural *s*), stop teaching that exemplar.
- **When to teach the next exemplar.** When you stop teaching one exemplar, move on to teaching the next exemplar. That is, when the child gives 10 consecutively, correct responses on one exemplar (e.g., "two books" in teaching the regular plural *s*), initiate treatment on the next exemplar (e.g., "two cats").
- **When to probe for generalized productions.** Probe as soon as you have taught 6 to 8 exemplars, each to the criterion of 10 consecutively correct, evoked responses.
- **When to go back to training more exemplars.** When the child's correct production of the target skills on probe exemplars falls short of the probe criterion (90% correct or 9 out of 10 correct probe responses), teach additional exemplars taken from the list of baserated exemplars.
- **When to consider a particular skill mastered.** When the child produces the target skill (e.g., the regular plural *s*) in new linguistic contexts and in conversational speech produced in naturalistic social situations (e.g., home, school), consider the skill as mastered.
- **When to initiate training on a new skill.** When the child meets the probe criterion for a given skill (e.g., the regular plural *s*), initiate training on a new skill (e.g., present progressive *ing*).
- **When to shift training to a higher level of response complexity.** When the child meets the probe criterion for a given level (e.g., the regular *s* in words), shift training to

the phrase or sentence level; note that, as mentioned in the previous bullet, you have the option of introducing a new skill as well.

In essence, the clinician initially baserates the target skill with multiple exemplars, teaches several exemplars, probes to see if the skill is generalized, offers treatment on additional exemplars if the probe criterion is not met, and probes again. Training and probing are alternated until the child meets the probe criterion (90% correct responses when untrained stimuli are presented). The child is dismissed from treatment when all the target skills needed for that child are taught with multiple exemplars and the child has met the probe criterion for each skill.

Initially, the clinician may select one or just a few target skills to teach in a given session. Most skills taught may be at the basic level—perhaps the word or phrase level. In subsequent sessions, the clinician may teach multiple skills, each at a different level. For instance, the clinician may begin teaching the regular plural *s*, the present progressive *ing*, and the preposition *on*—all in two-word phrases. Soon, the child may meet the training criterion for 6 to 8 exemplars of the plural *s* while still needing additional treatment for the other targets. Therefore, the clinician may shift training on the plural *s* to the sentence level while continuing to teach the other targets at the phrase level. Eventually, the clinician may be teaching different skills at vastly different levels (some at the phrase, others at the simple sentence, and still others at the extended sentence levels).

Providing Effective Feedback

The most critical treatment variable is effective and functional feedback. Children in treatment sessions need precise and prompt information on how they are doing. The protocols suggest verbal praise—a form of social reinforcement—as the most easily administered positive reinforcer for correct responses. Verbal praise is natural, inherent to most communicative situations, and can be delivered as soon as the child gives a correct response. It is known to be effective, and it does not cost anything. Children rarely get tired of honest verbal praise offered when their performance meets certain standards.

A reinforcer is effective and functional only when it results in an increased rate of responses for which it is being offered. Therefore, clinicians need to have options in case verbal praise proves ineffective with a child. With most children, a good option is the token system of reinforcement. Tokens are known as *conditioned generalized reinforcers* because they may be exchanged for a variety of reinforcers. The clinician may give a token for every correct response and let the child exchange the tokens for a small gift (the backup reinforcer) at the end of the session. Clinicians may also use such primary reinforcers as food items, but this requires a clearance from the parents and selection of healthful edibles.

Corrective feedback for incorrect responses is equally important. Children may be simply told that the response was incorrect or that something specified was missing. Even a statement of what the child should have said instead of what was said may be effective corrective feedback. Children readily accept corrective feedback when it is fair, delivered objectively, and immediately followed by helpful modeling or repetition of a trial on which the child succeeds. Although verbal corrective feedback is most commonly used—and hence it is a part of the protocols, there are other forms in case the need arises. Token withdrawal is an effective strategy that may be combined with verbal corrective feedback.

The clinician who awards a token for a correct response may withdraw one for an incorrect response. This strategy is known as *response cost.*

Excessive need to offer corrective feedback implies some problem with the treatment procedure. Perhaps the target skill needs to be simplified; maybe another target is suitable. The clinician may have to shape the child's behavior in small steps, so that the child experiences success at each step. This strategy helps avoid excessive or perhaps detrimental use of corrective feedback.

As the correct responses increase during treatment, the need for corrective feedback will automatically diminish. This situation, however, may result in an excessive and somewhat unnatural amount of positive reinforcement. The amount of reinforcement offered to a child should eventually approach what is typically offered in social situations. Therefore, the clinician should start with reinforcing every response (continuous reinforcement) and gradually move to an intermittent reinforcement schedule in which every second, third, or fourth response is correctly reinforced. This is easily accomplished when training moves to conversational speech in which the clinician only occasionally reinforces correct responses.

Measuring the Child's Progress

Clinicians appreciate the necessity of documenting the progress children (or adult clients) make in treatment sessions. This is especially critical for third-party payers. Regardless of payment issues, measurement of skills being taught is a necessary scientific task. The protocols make it easier to track children's responses during treatment so that clinicians have precise quantitative information that they can analyze in relation to the baserates. Virtually everything clinicians teach is quantifiable; if the client's responses are not quantified, no one can be sure what is going on in treatment.

The recording sheets available on the CD can be individualized for the clinic, the clinician, and the child. Diligently used, these recording sheets will give precise numbers of correct and incorrect responses a child gives in baserate, treatment, and probe sessions. The clinician thus will have precise and objective data to document a child's progress. For example, a child's baserate production of a particular grammatic morpheme may be at 10%; but it may increase to 90% or better during treatment; and may meet the 90% probe criterion at the end of treatment. Such quantitative data help quell any doubts about the need for treatment and the improvement that did take place as a result of treatment.

Part I
Functional Words, Phrases, and Sentences

Protocols for Teaching Functional Words, Phrases, and Sentences

Overview

Children produce their first words between 8 months to 16 months, although typically around the first birthday (Gleason, 2001; McLaughlin, 1998). A majority of first words children produce are names of objects and people around them. The words may be classified into animals, adjectives, kinship terms, furniture and household objects, food, and clothing. Soon the names of toys and affective terms become part of the expanding vocabulary.

Words are soon expanded into two-word phrases, which are progressively expanded into simple and then more complex sentences. Most children with a language disorder need to learn certain basic or more advanced words; the more severe the disorder, the greater the need to teach simple and basic words. Many children with language disorders may produce a set of basic words, but may fail to combine them into phrases and sentences. In any case, the clinician should be prepared to start teaching at the level the child fails to express. For some children, it might be the word level; for others, it might be the phrase or simple sentence level.

General Training Strategy

Teaching a set of functional words, phrases, and sentences is always a good starting point of language treatment. The general training strategy is to select child-specific words that are especially meaningful for the child in his or her family, social, and academic communication. The protocols that follow provide a set of words, but clinicians are encouraged to substitute child-specific words. For instance, the names of family members, pets, and favorite foods and activities are more relevant than generic terms. In that sense, the clinicians should find the words, phrases, and sentences given in this section as only suggestive of child-specific targets. In addition to the suggested words within the protocols, Appendix A provides a list of first few functional words children learn to produce. The clinician may select words from this list as well.

The clinician may baserate the production of some 20 functional words with the help of pictures or objects. Baserates provide a basis to compare the child's progress in treatment sessions. In any treatment session, the clinician may concentrate on teaching 6 to 8 words. The discrete trial procedure is effective in teaching words, phrases, and most morphologic features. Therefore, the protocols include the discrete trial procedure. Instructions, demonstrations, modeling, prompting, fading, and positive reinforcement for imitated and spontaneous responses and corrective feedback for incorrect responses constitute the main treatment techniques.

The clinician begins teaching with modeling; fades modeling as the child gives 5 consecutively correct imitated responses; reinstates modeling if the child fails to give correct responses on 3 to 4 trials on evoked trials. The clinician fades the modeling again as the child gives 5 consecutively correct imitated responses.

After teaching 6 to 8 words to a training criterion of 90% correct, the clinician administers a probe with different pictures that represent each target word (e.g., a different colored ball, a cup of different size, a hat of different shape and size, etc.).

If the child fails to meet the probe criterion of 90% correct, the clinician administers additional teaching trials on the already trained stimuli; subsequently, readministers the probe trials; and uses this teach-probe-teach strategy until the child meets the probe criterion.

When the child meets the probe criterion of 90% correct, the clinician either teaches new words or teaches phrases that are formed out of the previously taught words.

To teach the skills on discrete trials and to document the child's progress, the clinician may reproduce the baserate, treatment, and probe recording sheets given in the Appendixes or print them from the CD.

Functional Words

Baserate Protocols

On each trial, place a picture that represents the target word in front of the child and ask the question. Administer the evoked trials first followed by modeled trials. Do not provide feedback on any trials; just record the responses on the recording sheet provided on the next page (or printed from the CD).

Scripts for Evoked Baserate Trial		Note
Clinician	[Shows the picture of a ball] "What is this?"	No modeling.
Child	[says nothing]	Scored as a wrong response
Clinician	Pulls the picture toward her and records the response.	No corrective feedback
Clinician	[Shows the picture of a cup] "What is this?"	Next trial
Child	"Cup."	A correct response
Clinician	Pulls the picture toward her and records the response.	No verbal praise

Administer the modeled baserate trials only after completing the evoked trials on all 20 (or more) words.

Scripts for Modeled Baserate Trial		Note
Clinician	[Shows the picture of a dog] "What is this? Say, *dog.*"	Modeling
Child	[says nothing]	Scored as a wrong response
Clinician	Pulls the picture toward her and records the response.	No corrective feedback
Clinician	[Shows the picture of an apple] "What is this? Say, *apple.*"	Modeling
Child	"Apple."	A correct response
Clinician	Pulls the picture toward her and records the response.	No verbal praise

Functional Words

Exemplars and Baserate Recording Sheet

Print this page from the CD or photocopy this page for your clinical use.

Name/Age:	Date:
Goal: To establish the baserates of functional single word productions when asked "What is this?" while showing a picture or object.	Clinician:

Functional Words	Evoked	Modeled
1. doll		
2. car		
3. train		
4. bike		
5. phone (telephone)		
6. cookie		
7. apple		
8. banana		
9. cake		
10. candy		
11. socks		
12. shoes		
13. hat		
14. house		
15. chair		
16. table		
17. dog		
18. cat		
19. fish		
20. bird		
Percent correct baserate		

*See **Appendix A** for a list of additional words that children initially learn and select words from that list if desirable.*

After establishing the baserates, initiate treatment. Use the protocols that follow.

Functional Words

Treatment Protocols

Place a picture in front of the child and follow the protocols. On each trial, present the stimulus and point to it.

Scripts for Modeled Discrete Trial Training		Note
Clinician	[Presents the picture of a doll] "What is this? Say, **doll**."	Vocal emphasis on the target word
Child	[says nothing]	Scored as a wrong response
Clinician	[Re-presents the stimulus] "What is this? Say, **doll**."	Next trial
Child	"Doll."	A correct response
Clinician	"Very good! That is a doll!"	Verbal praise

Repeat the trials until the child gives 5 consecutively correct, imitated responses. When the child imitates 5 correct responses in sequence, fade the modeling. Each time, present the stimulus and point to it.

Scripts for Fading the Modeling		Note
Clinician	[Presents the picture of a doll] "This is a *doll*. What is this? Say, . . . "	Correct response modeled before the question
Child	[Looks puzzled]	Scored as a wrong response
Clinician	[Re-presents the picture of a doll] "This is a *doll*. What is this? Say, . . . "	Next trial
Child	"Doll."	A correct response; repeat these trials a few times
Clinician	"Very good! You said *doll*!!"	Verbal praise
Clinician	[Presents the picture of a doll] "What is this?"	All cues faded; **an evoked trial**
Child	"Doll"	A correct response
Clinician	"Excellent! You said *doll*!"	Verbal praise; repeat evoked trials until the child gives 10 consecutively correct responses. Teach another baserated word.

Functional Words

Exemplars and Treatment Recording Sheet

Print this page from the CD or photocopy this page for your clinical use.

Teach 6 to 8 words in initial sessions, using the previous scripts. Change the target words given in the recording sheet to suit the individual child.

Name/Age:	Date:
Goal: Production of single words with 90% accuracy when asked "What is this?" while showing a picture or object.	Clinician:

Clinician's Comments:

Scoring: Correct: ✓   Incorrect or no response: X

Target skills	Discrete Trials														
	1	2	3	4	5	6	7	8	9	10	11	12	13	14	15
1. doll															
2. car															
3. train															
4. bike															
5. phone															
6. cookie															
7. apple															
8. banana															

Teach 6 to 8 words each to a tentative training criterion of 10 consecutively correct nonimitated (evoked) responses. Then, conduct a probe to assess generalized productions (see next page). When the child meets the 90% correct probe criterion, teach new words. Use a general treatment recording sheet (Appendix C or print the page from the CD) to record the child's responses on training trials. Type in the new target words on the recording sheet.

Each time you teach 6 to 8 new words, conduct a probe to assess generalized production using varied pictures that represent the same target word.

Functional Words

Probe Protocols and Recording Sheet

Print this page from the CD or photocopy this page for your clinical use.

Find different pictures for the 6 to 8 trained words that have met the tentative training criterion of 10 consecutively correct responses on evoked trials. For instance, for the trained word doll, *select at least pictures of three (3) dolls that are different in size, color, or other distinguishing features. Present each probe doll picture on a separate probe trial. When the child meets the 90% correct probe response rate, select new words for training.*

If the child fails to meet the probe criterion on untrained pictures of varied stimuli, give 4 to 6 training trials on each of the probed stimuli. Then find additional and varied stimuli to readminister a probe. Alternate probes and treatment until the probe criterion is met.

Scripts for Probe Trials

Clinician	[Presents a varied trained stimulus of a *doll*] "What is this?"	No modeling or prompts
Child	"Doll."	A correct probe response to a new, different picture of the same trained object.
Clinician	[Does not respond to the child's production; records the response as correct.]	If the child were to give an incorrect response or fail to give any kind of a response, the clinician scores it as incorrect and gives no corrective feedback.

Name/Age:	Date:
Clinician:	**Session #:**
Target Behavior: Functional words (probes)	
Trained and Untrained Stimuli	**Score: + correct; – incorrect or no responses**
1. doll (UT: a different kind)	
2. car (UT: a different kind)	
3. train (UT: a different kind)	
4. bike (UT: a different kind)	
5. phone (UT: a different kind)	
6. cookie (UT: a different kind)	
7. apple (UT: a different kind)	
8. banana (UT: a different kind)	

UT = untrained, novel stimulus that may represent the same trained response (e.g., a different-looking doll or car than the one used in teaching).

When the child meets the 90% correct probe criterion, select new words for teaching. When you have a set of functional words (perhaps 25 to 50), teach phrases created out of one trained noun and an untrained (novel) word, perhaps an adjective (e.g., big ball, red apple, long train).

See the next page for suggested functional phrases.

Functional Phrases

Exemplars and Baserate Protocols

Print this page from the CD or photocopy this page for your clinical use.

Change the phrases to suit the individual child. Add new targets as found necessary.

There may be no need to baserate phrase productions in a child who has just learned to produce the target words. If you wish to baserate, however, use this sheet to record the responses on a set of evoked and a set of modeled trials.

Name/Age:	Date:
Goal: To establish baserate productions of functional phrases with 90% accuracy when asked "What is this?" while showing a picture or object.	Clinician:

Functional Phrases	Evoked	Modeled
1. pretty doll		
2. blue car		
3. long train		
4. red bike		
5. tiny phone (telephone)		
6. yummy cookie		
7. green apple		
8. yellow banana		
9. chocolate cake		
10. sweet candy		
11. white socks		
12. black shoes		
13. small hat		
14. big house		
15. green chair		
16. dining table		
17. nice dog		
18. baby cat		
19. blue fish		
20. red bird		
Percent correct baserate		

After establishing the baserates, initiate treatment. Use the protocols that follow.

Functional Phrases

Treatment Protocols

Place a picture in front of the child and follow the protocols. On each trial, present the stimulus and point to it.

Scripts for Modeled Discrete Trial Training		Note
Clinician	[Presents the picture of a doll] "What is this? Say, **pretty doll**."	Vocal emphasis on the target phrases
Child	"Doll."	A wrong response
Clinician	"True, it's a doll, but I want you to say, pretty doll."	Corrective feedback
Clinician	[Re-presents the stimulus] "What is this? Say, **pretty doll**."	Next trial
Child	"Pretty doll."	A correct response
Clinician	"Very good! That is a pretty doll, isn't it!"	Verbal praise

Repeat the trials until the child gives 5 consecutively correct, imitated responses. When the child imitates 5 correct responses in sequence, fade the modeling. Each time, present the stimulus and point to it.

Scripts for Fading the Modeling		Note
Clinician	[Presents the picture of a doll] "This is a pretty doll. What is this? Say, . . . "	Correct response modeled before the question
Child	[Looks puzzled]	Scored as a wrong response
Clinician	[Re-presents the picture of a doll] "This is a a *pretty doll*. What is this? Say, . . . "	Next trial
Child	"Pretty doll."	A correct response; repeat these trials a few times
Clinician	"Very good! You said *pretty doll*!!"	Verbal praise
Clinician	[Presents the picture of a doll] "What is this?"	All cues faded; **an evoked trial**
Child	"Pretty doll"	A correct response
Clinician	"Excellent! You said *pretty doll*!"	Verbal praise; repeat evoked trials until the child gives 10 consecutively correct responses. Teach another baserated word.

Functional Phrases

Exemplars and Treatment Recording Sheet

Print this page from the CD or photocopy this page for your clinical use.

Teach 6 to 8 words in initial sessions, using the previous scripts. Change the target words given in the recording sheet to suit the individual child.

Name/Age:	Date:
Goal: Production of phrases with 90% accuracy when asked "What is this?" while showing a picture or object.	Clinician:

Clinician's Comments:

Scoring: Correct: ✓   Incorrect or no response: X

Target skills	Discrete Trials														
	1	2	3	4	5	6	7	8	9	10	11	12	13	14	15
1. pretty doll															
2. blue car															
3. long train															
4. red bike															
5. tiny phone															
6. yummy cookie															
7. green apple															
8. yellow banana															

Teach 6 to 8 phrases each to a tentative training criterion of 10 consecutively correct nonimitated (evoked) responses. Then, conduct a probe to assess generalized productions (see next page). If you need to teach more phrases, copy the treatment recording sheet from Appendix C and type in the new phrases (or modify and print this page from the CD).

Each time you teach 6 to 8 new phrases, conduct a probe to assess generalized production using varied pictures that represent the same target phrase.

Functional Phrases

Probe Protocols and Recording Sheet

Print this page from the CD or photocopy this page for your clinical use.

Find different pictures for the 6 to 8 trained phrases that have met the tentative training criterion of 10 consecutively correct responses on evoked trials. For instance, for the trained phrase pretty doll, select at least pictures of three (3) dolls that are different in size, color, or other distinguishing features. Present each probe doll picture on a separate probe trial. When the child meets the 90% correct probe response rate, select new phrases for training.

If the child fails to meet the probe criterion on untrained pictures of varied stimuli, give 4 to 6 training trials on each of the probed stimuli. Then find additional and varied stimuli to readminister a probe. Alternate probes and treatment until the probe criterion is met.

Scripts for Probe Trials

Clinician	[Presents a varied trained stimulus of a *pretty doll*] "What is this?"	No modeling or prompts
Child	"Pretty Doll."	A correct probe response to a new, different picture of the same trained object.
Clinician	[Does not respond to the child's response; records the response as correct.]	If the child were to give an incorrect response or fail to give any kind of a response, the clinician scores it as incorrect and gives no corrective feedback.

Name:	Date:	Session #:
Age:	**Clinician:**	
Disorder: Language	**Target Behavior: Functional phrases (Probe)**	

Trained and Untrained Stimuli	Score: + correct; − incorrect or no responses
1. pretty doll (UT: a different kind)	
2. blue car (UT: a different kind)	
3. long train (UT: a different kind)	
4. red bike (UT: a different kind)	
5. tiny phone (UT: a different kind)	
6. yummy cookie (UT: a different kind)	
7. green apple (UT: a different kind)	
8. yellow banana (UT: a different kind)	

UT = Untrained, novel stimulus that may represent the same trained response (e.g., a different-looking doll or car than the one used in teaching).

When the child meets the 90% correct probe criterion, select new phrases for teaching. When you have taught a set of functional phrases (perhaps 40 to 50), teach sentences created out of trained plus new words (e.g., this is a big ball, I see a red apple, that is a long train).

Functional Sentences (Production)

Exemplars and Baserate Recording Sheet

Print this page from the CD or photocopy this page for your clinical use.

Change the sentences to suit the individual child. Add new targets as found necessary.

There may be no need to baserate sentence productions in a child who has just learned to produce phrases. If you wish to baserate, however, use this sheet to record the responses on a set of evoked and a set of modeled trials.

Name/Age:	Date:
Goal: To establish baserate productions of functional sentences when asked "What do you see?" while showing a picture or object.	Clinician:

Clinician's Comments:

Functional Phrases	Evoked	Modeled
1. I see a pretty doll		
2. I see a blue car		
3. I see a long train		
4. I see a red bike		
5. I see a tiny phone (telephone)		
6. I see a yummy cookie		
7. I see a green apple		
8. I see a yellow banana		
9. I see a chocolate cake		
10. I see a sweet candy		
11. I see a white sock		
12. I see a black shoe		
13. I see a small hat		
14. I see a big house		
15. I see a green chair		
16. I see a dining table		
17. I see a nice dog		
18. I see a baby cat		
19. I see a blue fish		
20. I scc a rcd bird		
Percent correct baserate		

After establishing the baserates, initiate treatment. Use the protocols that follow.

Functional Sentences (Production)

Treatment Protocols

Use the selected stimulus material to evoke speech in semicontrolled interactions.

Scripts for Modeled Sentence Production		Note
Clinician	[Shows a large picture of a story scene in a story book] "What do you see here?" Say, ***I see a pretty doll***."	Vocal emphasis on the target word
Child	"Pretty doll."	Scored as a wrong response
Clinician	"Yes, but I want you to say the whole sentence, *I see a pretty doll*."	Corrective feedback
Clinician	[Points to the target stimulus] "What do you see here? Say, ***I see a pretty doll***."	Next trial
Child	"I see a pretty doll."	A correct response
Clinician	"Very good! You do see a pretty doll!"	Verbal praise

Repeat the trials until the child gives 5 consecutively correct, imitated responses. When the child imitates 5 correct responses in sequence, fade the modeling. Each time, present the stimulus and point to it.

Scripts for More Spontaneous Conversation		Note
Clinician	[Points to the target stimulus] "You see a pretty doll here. What do you see here? Say, . . . "	Correct response modeled before the question
Child	"Pretty doll"	A wrong response
Clinician	"Yes, but I want you to say the whole sentence, like you did before."	Corrective feedback
Clinician	[Points to the target stimulus] "You see a pretty doll here. What do you see here? Say, . . . "	Next trial
Child	"I see a pretty doll."	A correct response; repeat these trials a few times
Clinician	"Very good! You said the whole sentence!"	Verbal praise
Clinician	[Points to the target stimulus] "What do you see here?"	All cues faded; **an evoked trial**
Child	"I see a pretty doll"	A correct response
Clinician	"Excellent! You said the whole sentence!"	Verbal praise; repeat evoked trials until the child gives 10 consecutively correct responses. Teach other sentences.

Functional Sentences (Production)

Exemplars and Treatment Recording Sheet

Print this page from the CD or photocopy this page for your clinical use.

Teach 6 to 8 sentences in initial sessions, using the previous scripts. Change the target sentences given in this recording sheet to suit the individual child.

Name/Age:	Date:
Goal: Production of sentences with 90% accuracy when asked "What do you see?" while showing a picture or object.	Clinician:

Clinician's Comments:

Scoring: Correct: ✓   Incorrect or no response: X

Target skills	Discrete Trials														
	1	2	3	4	5	6	7	8	9	10	11	12	13	14	15
1. I see a pretty doll															
2. I see a blue car															
3. I see a long train															
4. I see a red bike															
5. I see a tiny phone															
6. I see a yummy cookie															
7. I see a green apple															
8. I see a yellow banana															

Teach 6 to 8 sentences each to a tentative training criterion of 10 consecutively correct nonimitated (evoked) responses. Then, conduct a probe to assess generalized productions (see next page).

When the child meets the 90% correct probe criterion, teach new sentences. Type in the new target sentences on the general treatment recording sheet provided in Appendix C (or modify and print this page from the CD).

Each time you teach 6 to 8 new sentences, conduct a probe to assess generalized production using varied pictures that represent the same target word.

Functional Sentences (Production)

Probe Protocols and Recording Sheet

Print this page from the CD or photocopy this page for your clinical use.

Find different pictures for the 6 to 8 trained sentences that have met the tentative training criterion of 10 consecutively correct responses on evoked trials. For instance, for the trained sentence I see a pretty doll, *select of at least three (3) dolls that are different in size, color, or other distinguishing features. Present each probe picture on a separate probe trial. When the child meets the 90% correct probe response rate, select new sentences for training.*

If the child fails to meet the probe criterion on untrained pictures of varied stimuli, give 4 to 6 training trials on each of the probed stimuli. Then find additional and varied stimuli to readminister a new probe. Alternate probes and treatment until the probe criterion is met.

Scripts for Probe Trials

Clinician	[Presents a varied trained stimulus of a *pretty doll*] "What do you see here?"	No modeling or prompts
Child	"I see a pretty doll."	A correct probe response on a new, different picture of the same trained object
Clinician	Does not respond to the child's production; records the response as correct.	If the child were to give an incorrect response or fail to give any kind of a response, the clinician scores it as incorrect, and gives no corrective feedback

Name:	Date:	Session #:	
Age:	**Clinician:**		
Disorder: Language	**Target Behavior: Functional sentences (Probe)**		
Untrained Stimuli			**Score: + correct; – incorrect or no responses**
1. pretty doll (UT: a different kind) "I see a pretty doll."			
2. blue car (UT: a different kind) "I see a blue car."			
3. long train (UT: a different kind) "I see a long train."			
4. red bike (UT: a different kind) "I see a red bike."			
5. tiny phone (UT: a different kind) "I see a tiny phone."			
6. yummy cookie (UT: a different kind) "I see a yummy cookie."			
7. green apple (UT: a different kind) "I see a green apple."			
8. yellow banana (UT: a different kind) "I see a yellow banana."			

UT = Untrained, novel stimulus that may represent the same trained response (e.g., a different-looking doll or car than the one used in teaching).

When the child meets the 90% correct probe criterion, select new sentences for teaching. When you have taught a set of functional sentences, initiate training on morphologic features.

Part II

Morphologic Features

Protocols for Teaching Morphologic Features

Overview of Morphologic Features

- Morphologic features are part of the English grammar. Such small elements of language as the inflections (the regular plural, the past tense, and the possessive), irregular plurals and the past tense words, the present progressive *ing*, auxiliaries and copulas in their contractible and uncontractible forms, prepositions, pronouns, third person singular, and so forth are English morphologic features.
- A hallmark of language disorders in children is the omission or misuse of morphologic features. Virtually all children with language disorders need to be taught the morphologic features. Most morphologic features are essential to expand phrases into sentences and to expand language skills in general.

General Training Strategy

- Select 20 exemplars for each target morpheme
- Use the exemplars given for each morpheme in this section; add or delete additional exemplars to suit the child
- Select pictures or objects to represent the exemplars
- Baserate the production of each morpheme with the 20 exemplars selected; administer one set of modeled and one set of evoked trials
- Begin teaching at the phrase level; if the child has difficulty, teach a few single words with the target morpheme (e.g., *hats*, *walking*, *Mommy's*, etc.)
- Start teaching with the discrete trial method
- Use instructions, demonstrations, modeling, prompting, fading, and positive reinforcement for imitated and spontaneous responses and corrective feedback for incorrect responses
- Begin each morphologic teaching with modeling; fade modeling as the child gives 5 consecutively correct imitated responses; reinstate modeling if the child fails to give correct responses on 3 to 4 trials on evoked trials
- Teach 6 to 8 target exemplars in any given session; increase or decrease the number depending on the child's performance
- After teaching 6 to 8 exemplars for a given morpheme (e.g., 6 to 8 words or phrases with the plural *s*) to a training criterion of 90% correct, administer a probe in which you present untrained stimulus items
- If the child fails to meet the probe criterion, teach 4 to 6 new exemplars; use this teach-probe-teach strategy until the child meets the probe criterion
- When the child meets the probe criterion of 90% correct, shift training to a higher level of response complexity or teach a different target skill
- Reproduce the given recording sheets or print them from the CD to initially teach the skills on discrete trials and to document the child's progress

Regular Plural Morphemes

Overview

Plurality in English is expressed through both regular and irregular morphemes. Irregular plural morphemes are whole words (e.g., *women*, *children*), and are often described as *free morphemes* as they can convey meaning by themselves. Regular plural morphemes, on the other hand, are suffixes to root words and are described as bound (they are bound to other whole words, as in *cups* or *oranges*). Standing alone, such bound morphemes as the regular plural *s* would not convey meaning.

The regular plural morpheme has three commonly used allomorphic variations: the plural *s* (e.g., *cups*), the plural *z* (e.g., *bags*), and the plural *ez* (e.g., *oranges*). Although all spelled with an *s* in print, they are phonetically different.

Children who are learning their language normally begin to produce the regular plurals relatively early. In Brown's (1973) longitudinal study of 3 children, the regular plural was ranked number 4 in reaching mastery. This mastery was achieved in Brown's stage II of syntactic development (between ages 27 and 30 months).

General Training Strategy

Some of the early child language treatment efficacy research has shown that children need to be taught the regular plural allomorphic variations separately (e.g., Guess & Baer, 1973; Guess, Sailor, Rutherford, & Baer, 1968). If not, the children who are taught one allomorphic variation (e.g., the plural *s*) will inappropriately generalize it to words that take another variation (e.g., the plural *z*). Therefore, protocols are provided for teaching each of the three standard variations of the regular plural morpheme.

It is generally sufficient to teach 6 to 8 exemplars to have the child produce the regular plural allomorph in the context of new or untrained words. However, generalized productions vary across children. Therefore, the clinician needs to teach a few exemplars, probe for generalization, and teach additional exemplars when generalized productions fall below the typical criterion of 90% correct in the context of new (untaught) words.

Regular Plural *s*
Regular Plural *s* in Phrases

Baserate Protocols

Children master the regular plural inflections relatively early. It is one of the early language targets to teach children with language disorders. It is appropriate to teach the plural inflections when the child has mastered a set of basic words, phrases, and sentences. See the target phrases for the *s* allomorph on the next page.

On each trial, place a picture of plural objects that help evoke the plural s in front of the child and follow the protocol. Administer the evoked trials first followed by modeled trials. Do not provide feedback on any trials; just record the child's responses on the recording sheet provided on the next page or printed from the CD.

Scripts for Evoked Baserate Trial		Note
Clinician	"What are these?"	No modeling
Child	"Two hat." ["Hat."]	A wrong response
Clinician	Pulls the picture toward her and records the response.	No corrective feedback
Clinician	"What are these?"	The next trial
Child	"Two blocks." ["Blocks."]	A correct response
Clinician	Pulls the picture toward her and records the response.	No verbal praise

Administer the modeled baserate trials only after completing the evoked trials on all 20 (or more) exemplars. Again, place the relevant picture in front of the child before starting each trial.

Scripts for Modeled Baserate Trial		Note
Clinician	"These are two hats. What are these? Say, *two hats.*"	Modeling
Child	"Two hat."	A wrong response
Clinician	Pulls the picture toward her and records the response.	No corrective feedback
Clinician	"These are two cats. What are these? Say, *two cats.*"	Modeling
Child	"Two cats."	A correct response
Clinician	Pulls the picture toward her and records the response.	No verbal praise

After establishing the baserates of plural z production in phrases, begin teaching them. Use the exemplars and the recording sheet given on the next page (print it from the CD).

Regular Plural *s* in Phrases

Exemplars and Baserate Recording Sheet

Print this page from the CD or photocopy this page for your clinical use.

Name/Age:	Date:
Goal: To establish baserate production of plural *s* in phrases when asked "What are these?" while showing pictures or objects.	Clinician:

Clinician's Comments:

Scoring: Correct: ✓   Incorrect or no response: X

Plural *s* in Phrases	Evoked	Modeled
1. two hats		
2. two blocks		
3. two boats		
4. two rats		
5. two books		
6. two cakes		
7. two ducks		
8. two trucks		
9. two cats		
10. two goats		
11. two hats		
12. two mats		
13. two plants		
14. two plates		
15. two pots		
16. two rabbits		
17. two cups		
18. two socks		
19. two snakes		
20. two trucks		
Percent correct baserate		

Replace or add exemplars as you see fit for a given child.

After establishing the baserates, begin teaching the regular plural s in phrases. Use the protocols that follow.

Regular Plural *s* in Phrases

Treatment Protocols

At the beginning of each trial, place two pictures in front of the child, one showing a single hat and the other showing two hats. Each time, point to the correct stimulus.

Scripts for Modeled Discrete Trial Training		Note
Clinician	"This is a hat. These are two hats. What are these? Say, *two hats*."	Vocal emphasis on the target morpheme
Client	"Two hat."	A wrong response
Clinician	"No, that is not correct. What are these? Say, *two hats*."	Corrective feedback; continued vocal emphasis on the *s*
Client	"Two hats."	A correct response
Clinician	"Very good! You said *two hats*, not *hat*!"	Verbal praise

Repeat the trials until the child gives 5 consecutively correct, imitated responses. When the child imitates 5 correct responses in sequence, fade the modeling. Each time, point to the correct stimulus. Always show a picture before asking a question.

Scripts for Fading the Modeling		Note
Clinician	"This is a hat. These are two hats. What are these? Say, *two . . .*"	Partial modeling only
Client	"Two hat."	A wrong response
Clinician	"No, that is not correct. What are these? Say, *two . . .*"	Corrective feedback and partial modeling
Client	"Two hats."	A correct response
Clinician	"Very good! You said *two hats*, not *hat*!"	Verbal praise
Clinician	"These are two hats. What are these?"	Reduced cues (*singular form* omitted)
Client	"Two hats." ["hats"]	Both the forms accepted
Clinician	"Excellent! You said *two hats*!"	Verbal praise
Clinician	"What are these?"	**An Evoked Trial**
Client	"Two hats."	Typically correct answer

If the wrong responses persist on 4 to 5 evoked trials, reinstate partial or full modeling for a few trials, again fade the modeling, and re-present the evoked trials.

When the child meets the tentative learning criterion of 10 consecutively correct, nonimitated responses for a given stimulus item, move on to the next stimulus item. With this procedure, teach 6 to 8 exemplars shown on the following recording sheet. Use different exemplars as you see fit for a given child. Use the exemplars and the recording sheet given on the next page (or copy it from the CD).

Regular Plural *s* in Phrases

Exemplars and Treatment Recording Sheet

Print this page from the CD or photocopy this page for your clinical use.

Teach 6 to 8 exemplars using the previous scripts.

Name/Age:	Date:
Goal: Production of the plural *s* in phrases with 90% accuracy when asked "What are these?" while showing pictures or objects.	Clinician:

Clinician's Comments:

Scoring: Correct: ✓   Incorrect or no response: X

Target skills	Discrete Trials														
	1	2	3	4	5	6	7	8	9	10	11	12	13	14	15
1. hat: two hats															
2. block: two blocks															
3. boat: two boats															
4. rat: two rats															
5. book: two books															
6. cake: two cakes															
7. duck: two ducks															
8. truck: two trucks															

Teach 6 to 8 exemplars each to a training criterion of 10 consecutively correct nonimitated responses. Because there is no need to probe for generalized productions at the phrase level, shift training to the sentence level. Baserate before initiating treatment.

Regular Plural *s* in Sentences

Baserate Protocols

At the beginning of each trial, place a relevant picture in front of the child. Point to the picture and then ask the specified question. Do not respond in any way to the child's correct, incorrect, or lack of responses.

Scripts for Evoked Baserate Trial		Note
Clinician	"What are these?"	No modeling; evoked trial
Child	"Two hat."	A wrong response
Clinician	Pulls the picture toward her and records the response.	No corrective feedback
Clinician	"What are these? Start with *these are . . .*"	Prompts the sentence
Child	"These are two blocks."	A correct response
Clinician	Pulls the picture toward her and records the response.	No verbal praise

Administer the modeled baserate trials only after completing the evoked trials on all 20 (or more) exemplars. Again, place a relevant picture in front of the child at the beginning of each trial and then ask the question.

Scripts for Modeled Baserate Trial		Note
Clinician	"What are these? Say, *these are two hats.*"	Modeled trial
Child	"Two hat."	A wrong response
Clinician	Pulls the picture toward her and records the response.	No corrective feedback
Clinician	"What are these? Say, *these are two cats.*"	Another modeled trial
Child	"These are two cats."	A correct response
Clinician	Pulls the picture toward her and records the response.	No verbal praise

Use the exemplars given on the next page to establish the baserates of plural s *in sentences.*

Regular Plural s in Sentences

Exemplars and Baserate Recording Sheet

Print this page from the CD or photocopy this page for your clinical use.

Name/Age:	Date:
Goal: To establish the baserate production of the plural *s* in sentences when asked "What are these?" while showing pictures or objects.	Clinician:

Clinician's Comments:

Scoring: Correct: ✓   Incorrect or no response: X

Plural *s* in Sentences	Evoked	Modeled
1. These are two bats.		
2. These are two blocks.		
3. These are two boats.		
4. These are two books.		
5. These are two boots.		
6. These are two cats.		
7. These are two cups.		
8. These are two ducks.		
9. These are two gifts.		
10. These are two goats.		
11. These are two hats.		
12. These are two mats.		
13. These are two plants.		
14. These are two plates.		
15. These are two rabbits.		
16. These are two rats.		
17. These are two rocks.		
18. These are two shirts.		
19. These are two snakes.		
20. These are two trucks.		
Percent correct baserate		

Replace or add new exemplars as you see fit for a given child. After establishing the baserates of plural s *in sentences, begin teaching its production. Follow the protocols given on the next page.*

Regular Plural *s* in Sentences

Treatment Protocols

Teach 6 to 8 sentences with the plural s *using the following script.*

Place a picture showing plural objects (e.g., two hats) in front of the child. Each time, point to the correct stimulus.

Scripts for Modeled Discrete Trial Training		Note
Clinician	"What are these? Say, *these are two hats*."	Modeling; the target vocally emphasized
Child	"These are two hat."	A wrong response
Clinician	"No, that's not correct. you forgot the *s*.	Corrective feedback; the trial scored as incorrect
Clinician	What are these? Say, these are *two hats*."	The next trial
Child	"These are two hats."	A correct response
Clinician	"Excellent! You said the whole sentence correctly!"	Verbal praise

Repeat the trials until the child gives 5 consecutively correct, imitated responses. When the child imitates 5 correct responses in sequence, fade the modeling. Each time, present and point to the correct stimulus.

Scripts for Fading the Modeling		Note
Clinician	"What are these? Say, *these are two . . .*"	Partial modeling only
Child	"Hat."	Scored as a wrong response
Clinician	"No, that is not correct. You didn't say all of it and you forgot the *s*."	Corrective feedback; scored as incorrect
Clinician	What are these? Say, *these are two . . .*"	The next trial
Child	"These are two hats."	A correct response
Clinician	"Excellent! You said the whole sentence!"	Verbal praise
Clinician	"What are these?"	Typical question; **an evoked trial**
Child	"These are two hats."	A correct response

If the wrong responses persist on 4 to 5 evoked trials, reinstate partial or full modeling for a few trials, again fade the modeling, and re-present the evoked trials.

When the child meets the tentative learning criterion of 10 consecutively correct, nonimitated responses, for a given stimulus item, move on to the next stimulus item. With this procedure, teach 6 to 8 exemplars shown on the following recording sheet. Use different exemplars as you see fit for a given child.

Regular Plural *s* in Sentences

Exemplars and Treatment Recording Sheet

Print this page from the CD or photocopy this page for your clinical use.

Name/Age:	Date:
Goal: Production of the plural *s* in sentences with 90% accuracy when asked "What are these?" while showing pictures or objects.	Clinician:

Clinician's Comments:

Scoring: Correct: ✓   Incorrect or no response: X

Target skills	Discrete Trials														
	1	2	3	4	5	6	7	8	9	10	11	12	13	14	15
1. hats: These are two hats															
2. blocks: These are two blocks															
3. boats: These are two boats															
4. rats: These are two rats															
5. books: These are two books															
6. cakes: These are two cakes															
7. ducks: These are two ducks															
8. trucks: These are two trucks															

When the child has met the learning criterion 10 consecutively correct, evoked (nonimitated) responses for each of the 6 to 8 target sentences, conduct a probe to see if the plural s production has generalized to previously baserated but untrained sentences.

If the probes do not meet the 90% correct criterion for untrained sentences, teach additional sentences and then probe again.

Regular Plural *s* in Sentences

Probe Protocols and Recording Sheet

Print this page from the CD or photocopy this page for your clinical use.

On the probes, present only the untrained exemplars (UT). When the child fails to meet the 90% correct probe criterion, either teach 2 to 4 new exemplars or give additional training trials on already trained stimuli. If needed, select new exemplars for probes. Probe at least 10 untrained exemplars. Alternate probes and treatment until the probe criterion is met.

Scripts for Probe Trials

Clinician	[Presents an untrained stimulus] "What are these?"	No modeling or prompts
Child	"These are two bats."	A correct, generalized response
Clinician	Scores the response as correct.	Offers no reinforcement
Clinician	[Presents another untrained stimulus] "What are these?"	The second probe trial
Child	"Two cup."	A wrong probe response
Clinician	Score the response as incorrect.	Offers no corrective feedback

Name:	Date:	Session #:
Age:	**Clinician:**	
Disorder: Language	**Target Behavior: Plural *s* in phrases (probe)**	
Untrained Stimuli	**Score: + correct; – incorrect or no responses**	
1. These are two bats. (UT)		
2. These are two cups. (UT)		
3. These are two cats. (UT)		
4. These are two mats. (UT)		
5. These are two plants. (UT)		
6. These are two rocks. (UT)		
7. These are two shirts. (UT)		
8. These are two snakes. (UT)		
9. These are two coats. (UT)		
10. These are two rocks. (UT)		
11. These are two plates. (UT)		
12. These are two gifts. (UT)		
Percent correct: (Criterion: 90%)		

If the child does not meet the probe criterion, give additional training on already trained sentences and subsequently readminister the probe trials. When the child meets the 90% correct probe criterion for plural s in sentences, shift training to other morphologic features or to conversational speech in which the plural s is monitored and reinforced.

Regular Plural *z*
Regular Plural *z* in Phrases
Baserate Protocols

Although affixed with an *s*, some regular plural words phonetically end with a /z/. If a singular word ends with a voiced sound (e.g., *bag*), the plural *s* added to it is pronounced as [z]. Research shows that children need to be taught the *z* allomorph separately. See the target phrases for the *z* allomorph on the next page.

On each trial, place a picture of plural objects designed to evoke the plural z in front of the child and follow the protocol. Administer the evoked trials first followed by modeled trials. Do not provide feedback on any trials; just record the responses on the recording sheet provided on the next page or printed from the CD.

Scripts for Evoked Baserate Trial		Note
Clinician	"What are these?"	No modeling
Child	"Two dog." ["dog"]	A wrong response
Clinician	Pulls the picture toward her and records the response.	No corrective feedback
Clinician	"What are these?"	The next trial
Child	"Two dolls." ["dolls"]	A correct response
Clinician	Pulls the picture toward her and records the response.	No verbal praise

Administer the modeled baserate trials only after completing the evoked trials on all 20 (or more) exemplars. Again, place the relevant picture in front of the child before starting each trial.

Scripts for Modeled Baserate Trial		Note
Clinician	"These are two dogs. What are these? Say, *two dogs.*"	Modeling
Child	"Two dog."	A wrong response
Clinician	Pulls the picture toward her and records the response.	No corrective feedback
Clinician	"These are two cats. What are these? Say, *two dolls.*"	Modeling
Child	"Two dolls."	A correct response
Clinician	Pulls the picture toward her and records the response.	No verbal praise

Use the exemplars and the recording sheet given on the next page (or print it from the CD).

Regular Plural z in Phrases

Exemplars and Baserate Recording Sheets

Print this page from the CD or photocopy this page for your personal use.

Name/Age:	Date:
Goal: To establish the baserates of plural z allomorph in phrases when asked "What are these?" while showing pictures or objects.	Clinician:

Clinician's Comments:

Scoring: Correct: ✓   Incorrect or no response: X

Plural z in Phrases	Evoked	Modeled
1. two dogs		
2. two dolls		
3. two balls		
4. two birds		
5. two bugs		
6. two trees		
7. two bags		
8. two trains		
9. two cars		
10. two keys		
11. two apples		
12. two bears		
13. two bells		
14. two lions		
15. two pies		
16. two shoes		
17. two spoons		
18. two stars		
19. two pigs		
20. two tigers		
Percent correct baserate		

Replace or add exemplars as you see fit for a given child. After you establish the baserates of plural z, begin teaching. Follow the protocols given on the next page.

Regular Plural *z* in Phrases

Treatment Protocols

At the beginning of each trial, place two pictures in front of the child, one showing a single dog and the other showing two dogs. Each time, point to the correct stimulus.

Scripts for Modeled Discrete Trial Training		Note
Clinician	"This is a dog. These are two dogs. What are these? Say, *two dog**s**.*"	Vocal emphasis on the target morpheme
Client	"Two dog."	A wrong response
Clinician	"No, that is not correct. What are these? Say, *two dog**s**.*"	Corrective feedback; continued vocal emphasis on the *z*
Client	"Two dogs."	A correct response
Clinician	"Very good! You said *two dog**s**, not *dog*!*"	Verbal praise

Repeat the trials until the child gives 5 consecutively correct, imitated responses. When the child imitates 5 correct responses in sequence, fade the modeling. Each time, point to the correct stimulus. Always show a picture before asking a question.

Scripts for Fading the Modeling		Note
Clinician	"This is a dog. These are two dogs. What are these? Say, *two . . .*"	Partial modeling only
Client	"Two dog."	A wrong response
Clinician	"No, that is not correct. What are these? Say, *two . . .*"	Corrective feedback and partial modeling
Client	"Two dogs."	A correct response
Clinician	"Very good! You said *two dog**s**, not *dog*!*"	Verbal praise
Clinician	"These are two dogs. What are these?"	Reduced cues (*singular form* omitted)
Client	"Two dogs." ["dogs"]	Both the forms accepted
Clinician	"Excellent! You said *two dog**s**!*"	Verbal praise
Clinician	"What are these?"	**An Evoked Trial**
Client	"Two dogs."	Typically correct answer

If the wrong responses persist on 4 to 5 evoked trials, reinstate partial or full modeling for a few trials, again fade the modeling, and re-present the evoked trials.

When the child meets the tentative learning criterion of 10 consecutively correct, nonimitated responses, for a given stimulus item, move on to the next stimulus item. With this procedure, teach 6 to 8 exemplars shown on the following recording sheet. Use different exemplars as you see fit for a given child. Use the exemplars and the recording sheet given on the next page (or print it from the CD).

Regular Plural z in Phrases

Exemplars and Treatment Recording Sheet

Print this page from the CD or photocopy this page for your clinical use.

Teach 6 to 8 exemplars using the previous scripts.

Name/Age:	Date:
Goal: Production of the plural allomorph z in phrases with 90% accuracy while showing pictures or objects.	Clinician:

Clinician's Comments:

Scoring: Correct: ✓   Incorrect or no response: X

Target skills	Discrete Trials														
	1	2	3	4	5	6	7	8	9	10	11	12	13	14	15
1. dog: two dogs															
2. doll: two dolls															
3. ball: two balls															
4. bird: two birds															
5. bug: two bugs															
6. tree: two trees															
7. bag: two bags															
8. train: two trains															

Teach 6 to 8 exemplars each to a training criterion of 10 consecutively correct nonimitated responses. Because there is no need to probe at the phrase level, shift training to the sentence level.

Regular Plural z in Sentences

Baserate Protocols

At the beginning of each trial, place a relevant picture in front of the child. Point to the picture and then ask the specified question. Do not respond in any way to the child's correct, incorrect, or lack of responses.

Scripts for Evoked Baserate Trial		Note
Clinician	"What are these?"	No modeling; evoked trial
Child	"Two dog."	A wrong response
Clinician	Pulls the picture toward her and records the response.	No corrective feedback
Clinician	"What are these? Start with *these are* . . ."	Prompts the sentence
Child	"These are two dogs."	A correct response
Clinician	Pulls the picture toward her and records the response.	No verbal praise

Administer the modeled baserate trials only after completing the evoked trials on all 20 (or more) exemplars. Again, place a relevant picture in front of the child at the beginning of each trial and then ask the question.

Scripts for Modeled Baserate Trial		Note
Clinician	"What are these? Say, *these are two dogs.*"	Modeled trial
Child	"Two dog."	A wrong response
Clinician	Pulls the picture toward her and records the response.	No corrective feedback
Clinician	"What are these? Say, *these are two dolls.*"	Another modeled trial
Child	"These are two dolls."	A correct response
Clinician	Pulls the picture toward her and records the response.	No verbal praise

Use the exemplars and the recording sheet given on the next page to establish the baserates of plural z in sentences (or print it from the CD).

Regular Plural z in Sentences

Exemplars and Baserate Recording Sheet

Print this page from the CD or photocopy this page for your clinical use.

Name/Age:		Date:
Goal: To establish the baserates of plural z in sentences when asked "What are these?" while showing pictures or objects.		Clinician:

Clinician's Comments:

Scoring: Correct: ✓   Incorrect or no response: X

Plural z in Sentences	Evoked	Modeled
1. These are two dogs.		
2. These are two dolls.		
3. These are two balls.		
4. These are two birds.		
5. These are two bugs.		
6. These are two trees.		
7. These are two bags.		
8. These are two trains.		
9. These are two cars.		
10. These are two keys.		
11. These are two apples.		
12. These are two bears.		
13. These are two bells.		
14. These are two lions.		
15. These are two pies.		
16. These are two shoes.		
17. These are two spoons.		
18. These are two stars.		
19. These are two pigs.		
20. These are two tigers		
Percent correct baserate		

Replace or add new exemplars as you see fit for a given child. After establishing the baserates of plural z in sentences, begin teaching its production. Follow the protocols given on the next page.

Regular Plural *z* in Sentences

Treatment Protocols

Teach 6 to 8 sentences with the plural z using the following script.

Place a picture in front of the child, showing plural objects (e.g., two dogs). Each time, point to the correct stimulus.

Scripts for Modeled Discrete Trial Training		Note
Clinician	"What are these? Say, *these are two dogs*."	Modeling; the target vocally emphasized
Child	"These are two dog." ["Two dogs."]	A wrong response
Clinician	"No, that's not correct. You forgot the **z** sound. ["No, you didn't say the whole sentence."]	Corrective feedback; the trial scored as incorrect
Clinician	What are these? Say, *these are two dogs*."	The next trial
Child	"These are two dogs."	A correct response
Clinician	"Excellent! You said the whole sentence correctly!"	Verbal praise

Repeat the trials until the child gives 5 consecutively correct, imitated responses. When the child imitates 5 correct responses in sequence, fade the modeling. Each time, present and point to the correct stimulus.

Scripts for Fading the Modeling		Note
Clinician	"What are these? Say, *these are two . . .*"	Partial modeling only
Child	"Dog."	Scored as a wrong response
Clinician	"No, that is not correct. You didn't say all of it and you forgot the *z* sound."	Corrective feedback; scored as incorrect
Clinician	What are these? Say, *these are two . . .*"	The next trial
Child	"These are two dogs."	A correct response
Clinician	"Excellent! You said the whole sentence!"	Verbal praise
Clinician	"What are these?"	Typical question; **an evoked trial**
Child	"These are two dogs."	A correct response

If the wrong responses persist on 4 to 5 evoked trials, reinstate partial or full modeling for a few trials, again fade the modeling, and re-present the evoked trials.

When the child meets the tentative learning criterion of 10 consecutively correct, nonimitated responses, for a given stimulus item, move on to the next stimulus item. With this procedure, teach 6 to 8 exemplars shown on the following recording sheet. Use different exemplars as you see fit for a given child.

Regular Plural z in Sentences

Exemplars and Treatment Recording Sheet

Print this page from the CD or photocopy this page for your clinical use.

Name/Age:	Date:
Goal: Production of the plural z in sentences with 90% accuracy when asked "What are these?" while showing pictures or objects.	Clinician:

Clinician's Comments:

Scoring: Correct: ✓   Incorrect or no response: X

Target skills	Discrete Trials														
	1	2	3	4	5	6	7	8	9	10	11	12	13	14	15
1. dogs: These are two dogs															
2. dolls: These are two dolls															
3. balls: These are two balls															
4. birds: These are two birds															
5. bugs: These are two bugs															
6. trees: These are two trees															
7. bags: These are two bags															
8. trains: These are two trains															

When the child has met the learning criterion of 10 consecutively correct, evoked (nonimitated) responses for each of the 6 to 8 target sentences, conduct a probe to see if the plural z production has generalized to previously baserated but untrained sentences. Use the protocols given on the next page (or print it from the CD).

Regular Plural z in Sentences

Probe Protocols and Recording Sheet

Print this page from the CD or photocopy this page for your clinical use.

On the probes, present only the untrained exemplars (UT). When the child fails to meet the 90% correct probe criterion, either teach 2 to 4 new exemplars or give additional training trials on already trained stimuli. If needed, select new exemplars for probes. Probe at least 10 untrained exemplars. Alternate probes and treatment until the probe criterion is met.

Scripts for Probe Trials

Clinician	[Presents an untrained stimulus] "What are these?"	No modeling or prompts
Child	"These are two cars."	A correct, generalized response
Clinician	Scores the response as correct.	Offers no reinforcement
Clinician	[Presents another untrained stimulus] "What are these?"	The second probe trial
Child	"Two key." ["These are two key."]	A wrong probe response
Clinician	Scores the response as incorrect.	Offers no corrective feedback

Name:	Date:	Session #:
Age:	**Clinician:**	
Disorder: Language	**Target Behavior: Plural z in sentences (probe)**	
Untrained Stimuli	**Score: + correct; – incorrect or no responses**	
1. These are two cars. (UT)		
2. These are two keys. (UT)		
3. These are two apples. (UT)		
4. These are two bears. (UT)		
5. These are two bells. (UT)		
6. These are two lions. (UT)		
7. These are two pies. (UT)		
8. These are two shoes. (UT)		
9. These are two spoons. (UT)		
10. These are two stars. (UT)		
11. These are two pigs. (UT)		
12. These are two tigers. (UT)		
Percent correct probe: (Criterion: 90%)		

If the child does not meet the probe criterion, give additional training on already trained sentences and subsequently readminister the probe trials. When the child meets the 90% correct probe criterion for plural z in sentences, shift training to other morphologic features or to conversational speech in which the plural z is monitored and reinforced.

Regular Plural *ez*
Regular Plural *ez* in Phrases
Baserate Protocols

Some plural words end with the *ez* morpheme, although orthographically they take the suffix *es*. These, too, have to be taught separately.

On each trial, place a picture of plural objects that help evoke the plural ez in front of the child and follow the protocol. Administer the evoked trials first followed by modeled trials. Do not provide feedback on any trials; just record the responses on the recording sheet provided on the next page or printed from the CD.

Scripts for Evoked Baserate Trial		Note
Clinician	"What are these?"	No modeling
Child	"Two box." ["box"]	A wrong response
Clinician	Pulls the picture toward her and records the response.	No corrective feedback
Clinician	"What are these?"	The next trial
Child	"Two dishes." ["dishes"]	A correct response
Clinician	Pulls the picture toward her and records the response.	No verbal praise

Administer the modeled baserate trials only after completing the evoked trials on all 20 (or more) exemplars. Again, place the relevant picture in front of the child before starting each trial.

Scripts for Modeled Baserate Trial		Note
Clinician	"These are two boxes. What are these? Say, *two boxes.*"	Modeling
Child	"Two box."	A wrong response
Clinician	Pulls the picture toward her and records the response.	No corrective feedback
Clinician	"These are two dishes. What are these? Say, *two dishes.*"	Modeling
Child	"Two dishes."	A correct response
Clinician	Pulls the picture toward her and records the response.	No verbal praise

Baserate at least 20 stimulus pictures as shown on the next page.

Regular Plural *ez* in Phrases

Exemplars and Baserate Recording Sheet

Print this page from the CD or photocopy this page for your clinical use.

Name/Age:	Date:
Goal: To establish the baserates of plural *ez* in phrases when asked "What are these?" while showing a picture or object.	Clinician:

Clinician's Comments:

Scoring: Correct: ✓   Incorrect or no response: X

Plural *ez* in Phrases	Evoked	Modeled
1. two boxes		
2. two dishes		
3. two houses		
4. two prizes		
5. two noses		
6. two buses		
7. two vases		
8. two foxes		
9. two dresses		
10. two houses		
11. two blouses		
12. two bridges		
13. two brushes		
14. two cages		
15. two horses		
16. two matches		
17. two oranges		
18. two peaches		
19. two watches		
20. two fences		
Percent correct baserate		

Replace or add exemplars as you see fit for the child.

After establishing the baserates of plural ez production in phrases, begin teaching them. Use the protocols given on the next page.

Regular Plural *ez* in Phrases

Treatment Protocols

At the beginning of each trial, place two pictures in front of the child (e.g., one showing a single box and the other showing two boxes). Each time, point to the correct stimulus.

Scripts for Modeled Discrete Trial Training		Note
Clinician	"This is a box. These are two boxes. What are these? Say, *two boxes*."	Vocal emphasis on the target morpheme
Client	"Two box."	A wrong response
Clinician	"No, that is not correct. What are these? Say, *two boxes*."	Corrective feedback; vocal emphasis on the *s*
Client	"Two boxes."	A correct response
Clinician	"Very good! You said *two boxes*, not *box*!"	Verbal praise

Repeat the trials until the child gives 5 consecutively correct, imitated responses. When the child imitates 5 correct responses in sequence, fade the modeling. Each time, point to the correct stimulus. Always show a picture before asking a question.

Scripts for Fading the Modeling		Note
Clinician	"This is a box. These are two boxes. What are these? Say, *two . . .*"	Partial modeling only
Client	"Two box."	A wrong response
Clinician	"No, that is not correct. What are these? Say, *two . . .*"	Corrective feedback and partial modeling
Client	"Two boxes."	A correct response
Clinician	"Very good! You said *two boxes*, not *box*!"	Verbal praise
Clinician	"These are two boxes. What are these?"	Reduced cues (singular form omitted)
Client	"Two boxes." ["boxes"]	Both the forms accepted
Clinician	"Excellent! You said *two boxes*!"	Verbal praise
Clinician	"What are these?"	**An Evoked Trial**
Client	"Two boxes."	Typically correct answer

If the wrong responses persist on 4 to 5 evoked trials, reinstate partial or full modeling for a few trials, again fade the modeling, and re-present the evoked trials.

When the child meets the tentative learning criterion of 10 consecutively correct, nonimitated responses for a given stimulus item, move on to the next stimulus item. With this procedure, teach 6 to 8 exemplars using the recording sheet shown on the following page. Use different exemplars as you see fit for a given child. Use the exemplars and the recording sheet given on the next page (or print it from the CD).

Teaching the Regular Plural *ez* in Phrases

Exemplars and Treatment Recording Sheet

Print this page from the CD or photocopy this page for your clinical use.

Name/Age:	Date:
Goal: Production of the plural allomorph *ez* in phrases with 90% accuracy when asked "What are these?" while showing pictures or objects.	Clinician:

Clinician's Comments:

Scoring: Correct: ✓   Incorrect or no response: X

Target skills	Discrete Trials														
	1	2	3	4	5	6	7	8	9	10	11	12	13	14	15
1. box: two boxes															
2. dish: two dishes															
3. hose: two hoses															
4. prize: two prizes															
5. nose: two noses															
6. bus: two buses															
7. vase: two vases															
8. fox: two foxes															

Teach 6 to 8 exemplars each to a training criterion of 10 consecutively correct, evoked (nonimitated) responses. Because there is no need for probes at the phrase level, shift training to the sentence level.

Regular Plural *ez* in Sentences
Baserate Protocols

At the beginning of each trial, place a relevant picture in front of the child. Point to the picture and then ask the specified question. Do not respond in any way to the child's correct, incorrect, or lack of responses.

Scripts for Evoked Baserate Trial		Note
Clinician	"What are these?"	No modeling; evoked trial
Child	"Two box."	A wrong response
Clinician	Pulls the picture toward her and records the response.	No corrective feedback
Clinician	"What are these? Start with *these are . . .*"	Prompts the sentence
Child	"These are two boxes."	A correct response
Clinician	Pulls the picture toward her and records the response.	No verbal praise

Administer the modeled baserate trials only after completing the evoked trials on all 20 (or more) exemplars. Again, place a relevant picture in front of the child at the beginning of each trial and then ask the question.

Scripts for Modeled Baserate Trial		Note
Clinician	"What are these? Say, *these are two boxes.*"	Modeled trial
Child	"Two box."	A wrong response
Clinician	Pulls the picture toward her and records the response.	No corrective feedback
Clinician	"What are these? Say, *these are two dishes.*"	Another modeled trial
Child	"These are two dishes."	A correct response
Clinician	Pulls the picture toward her and records the response.	No verbal praise

Use the exemplars and the recording sheet given on the next page to establish the baserates of plural ez in sentences (or print it from the CD).

Regular Plural *ez* in Sentences

Exemplars and Baserate Recording Sheet

Print this page from the CD or photocopy this page for your clinical use.

Name/Age:	Date:
Goal: To establish the baserates of plural *ez* in sentences when asked "What are these?" while showing pictures or objects.	Clinician:

Clinician's Comments:

Scoring: Correct: ✓   Incorrect or no response: X

Sentence Level	Evoked	Modeled
1. These are two boxes.		
2. These are two dishes.		
3. These are two houses.		
4. These are two prizes.		
5. These are two noses.		
6. These are two buses.		
7. These are two vases.		
8. These are two foxes.		
9. These are two dresses.		
10. These are two houses.		
11. These are two blouses.		
12. These are two bridges.		
13. These are two brushes.		
14. These are two cages.		
15. These are two horses.		
16. These are two matches.		
17. These are two oranges.		
18. These are two peaches.		
19. These are two watches.		
20. These are two fences.		
Percent correct baserate		

Replace or add new exemplars as you see fit for a given child.

After establishing the baserates for the plural ez in sentences, initiate treatment. Use the protocols given on the next page.

Regular Plural *ez* in Sentences

Treatment Protocols

Teach 6 to 8 sentences with the plural ez using the following script.

Place a picture in front of the child, showing plural objects (e.g., two boxes). Each time, point to the correct stimulus.

Scripts for Modeled Discrete Trial Training		Note
Clinician	"What are these? Say, *these are two box**es**.*"	Modeling; the target vocally emphasized
Child	"These are two box." ["Two boxes"]	A wrong response
Clinician	"No, that's not correct. you forgot the **ez** sound. ["No, you didn't say the whole sentence."]	Corrective feedback; the trial scored as incorrect
Clinician	What are these? Say, *these are two box**es**.*"	The next trial
Child	"These are two boxes."	A correct response
Clinician	"Excellent! You said the whole sentence correctly!"	Verbal praise

Repeat the trials until the child gives 5 consecutively correct, imitated responses. When the child imitates 5 correct responses in sequence, fade the modeling. Each time, present and point to the correct stimulus.

Scripts for Fading the Modeling		Note
Clinician	"What are these? Say, *these are two . . .*"	Partial modeling only
Child	"Box."	Scored as a wrong response
Clinician	"No, that is not correct. You didn't say all of it and you forgot the *ez sound.*"	Corrective feedback; scored as incorrect
Clinician	What are these? Say, *these are two . . .*"	The next trial
Child	"These are two boxes."	A correct response
Clinician	"Excellent! You said the whole sentence!"	Verbal praise
Clinician	"What are these?"	Typical question; **an evoked trial**
Child	"These are two boxes."	A correct response

If the wrong responses persist on 4 to 5 evoked trials, reinstate partial or full modeling for a few trials, again fade the modeling, and re-present the evoked trials.

When the child meets the tentative learning criterion of 10 consecutively correct, nonimitated responses, for a given stimulus item, move on to the next stimulus item. With this procedure, teach 6 to 8 exemplars shown on the following recording sheet. Use different exemplars as you see fit for a given child.

Regular Plural *ez* in Sentences

Exemplars and Treatment Recording Sheet

Print this page from the CD or photocopy this page for your clinical use.

Name/Age:	Date:
Goal: Production of the plural *ez* in sentences with 90% accuracy when asked "What are these?" while showing pictures or objects.	Clinician:

Clinician's Comments:

Scoring: Correct: ✓   Incorrect or no response: X

Target skills	Discrete Trials														
	1	2	3	4	5	6	7	8	9	10	11	12	13	14	15
1. boxes: These are two boxes															
2. dishes: These are two dishes															
3. hoses: These are two hoses															
4. prizes: These are two prizes															
5. noses: These are two noses															
6. buses: These are two buses															
7. bags: These are two bags															
8. foxes: These are two foxes															

When the child has met the learning criterion of 10 consecutively correct, evoked (nonimitated) responses for each of the 6 to 8 target sentences, conduct a probe to see if the plural ez production has generalized to previously baserated but untrained sentences.

Use the protocols given on the next page (or, print it from the CD).

Regular Plural *ez* in Sentences
Probe Protocols and Recording Sheet

Print this page from the CD or photocopy this page for your clinical use.

On the probes, present only the untrained exemplars (UT). When the child fails to meet the 90% correct probe criterion, either teach 2 to 4 new exemplars or give additional training trials on already trained stimuli. If needed, select new exemplars for probes. Probe at least 10 untrained exemplars. Alternate probes and treatment until the probe criterion is met.

Scripts for Probe Trials

Clinician	[Presents an untrained stimulus] "What are these?"	No modeling or prompts
Child	"These are two dresses."	A correct, generalized response
Clinician	Scores the response as correct.	Offers no reinforcement
Clinician	[Presents another untrained stimulus] "What are these?"	The second probe trial
Child	"Two houses." ["These are two house."]	A wrong probe response
Clinician	Scores the response as incorrect.	Offers no corrective feedback

Name:	Date:	Session #:
Age:	**Clinician:**	
Disorder: Language	**Target Behavior: Plural *ez* in sentences (probe)**	
Untrained Stimuli	**Score: + correct; – incorrect or no responses**	
1 These are two dresses. (UT)		
2 These are two houses. (UT)		
3 These are two blouses. (UT)		
4. These are two bridges. (UT)		
5. These are two bushes. (UT)		
6. These are two cages. (UT)		
7. These are two horses. (UT)		
8. These are two matches. (UT)		
9. These are two oranges. (UT)		
10. These are two peaches. (UT)		
11. These are two watches. (UT)		
12. These are two fences. (UT)		
Percent correct probe (Criterion: 90%)		

If the child does not meet the probe criterion, give additional training on already trained sentences and subsequently readminister the probe trials. When the child meets the 90% correct probe criterion for plural ez in sentences, shift training to other morphologic features (such as irregular plurals as shown next) or to conversational speech in which the plural ez is monitored and reinforced.

Irregular Plural Words

Overview

- Irregular plural morphemes are whole words.
- Irregular plural words are not a single response class. This means that, unlike regular plural words, teaching a few irregular plurals will not result in the generalized production of other irregular plurals. Therefore, each irregular plural word is a separate treatment target.
- There are many irregular plurals—some infrequently used—but the clinician can make a judgment about their functionality and select some 20 relatively common words to teach. Some infrequently used irregular plural words (e.g., phenomena, data) may be important to teach children in view of their academic demands, however.

General Training Strategy

- The strategy for teaching irregular plurals is more similar to teaching functional words than it is to teach regular plural morphemes.
- Select 20 functional irregular plurals that are child-specific; begin with the words provided and add or delete words to suit the needs of individual children.
- Select pictures or objects to represent the exemplars.
- Baserate the production of each irregular plural on one set of evoked and another set of modeled trials.
- Teach 6 to 8 words in a session, using discrete trials; increase or decrease the number depending on the child's performance.
- Use instructions, demonstrations, modeling, prompting, fading, and positive reinforcement for imitated and spontaneous responses and corrective feedback for incorrect responses.
- Begin each target irregular plural word teaching with modeling; fade modeling as the child gives 5 consecutively correct, imitated responses; reinstate modeling if the child fails to give correct responses on 3 to 4 evoked trials.
- After teaching 6 to 8 irregular plural words, each to a training criterion of 90% correct, administer a probe with different pictures that represent each target word (e.g., pictures of different men, women, leaves, or fish).
- If the child fails to meet the probe criterion of 90% correct, administer additional teaching trials on the already trained stimuli; readminister the probe trials; use this teach-probe-teach strategy until the child meets the probe criterion.
- When the child meets the probe criterion of 90% correct, teach additional irregular plural words.
- Reproduce the recording sheets that follow or print them from the CD to teach the skills on discrete trials and to document the child's progress.

Irregular Plural Words
Irregular Plural Words in Phrases
Baserate Protocols

On each trial, place a picture that represents the target plural word (e.g., two women) in front of the child and ask the question. Administer the evoked trials first followed by modeled trials. Do not provide feedback on any trials; just record the child's responses on the recording sheet provided on the next page (or printed from the CD).

Scripts for Evoked Baserate Trial		Note
Clinician	[*Shows the picture of two women*] "Who are these?"	No modeling
Child	[says nothing]	Scored as a wrong response
Clinician	Pulls the picture toward her and records the response.	No corrective feedback
Clinician	[*Shows the picture of two men*] "Who are these?"	Next trial
Child	"Men." ["Two men."]	A correct response
Clinician	Pulls the picture toward her and records the response.	No verbal praise

Administer the modeled baserate trials only after completing the evoked trials on all 20 (or more) words.

Scripts for Modeled Baserate Trial		Note
Clinician	[*Shows the picture of two women*] "Who are these? Say, *two women.*"	Modeling
Child	[says nothing]	Scored as a wrong response
Clinician	Pulls the picture toward her and records the response.	No corrective feedback
Clinician	[*Shows the picture of two men*] "Who are these? Say, *two men.*"	Modeling
Child	"Two men."	A correct response
Clinician	Pulls the picture toward her and records the response.	No verbal praise

Irregular Plural Words in Phrases

Exemplars and Baserate Recording Sheet

Print this page from the CD or photocopy this page for your clinical use.

Name/Age:	Date:
Goal: To establish the baserates of irregular plural words in phrases when asked "What are these?" while showing a picture or object.	Clinician:

Clinician's Comments:

Scoring: Correct: ✓   Incorrect or no response: X

Irregular Plural Words	Evoked	Modeled
1. woman: two women		
2. man: two men		
3. child: three children		
4. foot: two feet		
5. tooth: many teeth		
6. goose: four geese		
7. mouse: three mice		
8. sheep: two sheep		
9. fish: many fish		
10. deer: five deer		
11. dice: many dice		
12. moose: two moose		
13. calf: four calves		
14. loaf: two loaves		
15. wife: two wives		
16. leaf: many leaves		
17. wolf: three wolves		
18. knife: two knives		
19. ox: four oxen		
20. fungus: many fungi		
Percent correct baserate		

Replace or add exemplars as you see fit for a given child. After establishing the baserates, initiate treatment. Use the protocols given on the next page.

Irregular Plural Words in Phrases
Treatment Protocols

This protocol shows that to begin with, a clinician teaches irregular plurals in phrases. If the child has difficulty at the phrase level, teach a few single irregular words before moving on to phrases. Model single words (e.g., women) as against the phrase (e.g., two women).

Place the paired pictures (singular/plural representations) in front of the child and follow the protocols. On each trial, present the stimuli and point to the specific one.

Scripts for Modeled Discrete Trial Training		Note
Clinician	[Shows the paired stimuli] "This is one woman. These are two women. Who are these? Say, *two* **women**."	Vocal emphasis on the target word
Child	[says nothing]	Scored as a wrong response
Clinician	[*Re-presents the stimuli*] "This is one woman. These are two women. Who are these? Say, *two women*."	Next trial
Child	"Two woman."	An incorrect response
Clinician	"No, that's not correct. When you see more than one, you say, *women*."	Corrective feedback, rule explanation
Clinician	[*Re-presents the stimuli*] "This is one woman. These are two women. Who are these? Say, *two* **women**."	Increased vocal emphasis on the target word
Child	"Two women." ["women"]	A correct response
Clinician	"Very good! You said *women*, not *woman*!"	Verbal praise

Repeat the trials until the child gives 5 consecutively correct, imitated responses. When the child imitates 5 correct responses in sequence, fade the modeling. Each time, present the stimulus and point to it.

Scripts for Fading the Modeling		Note
Clinician	[*Shows the target stimulus*] "These are two women. Who are these? Say, *two* . . ."	Partial modeling; omits the singular form
Child	"Woman"	A wrong response
Clinician	"No, that's not correct. Remember, when you see more than one, you say, *women*."	Corrective feedback
Clinician	[*Re-presents the stimulus*] "These are two women. Who are these? Say, two . . ."	Next trial
Child	"Two women."	A correct response
Clinician	"Very good! You said *women*!!"	Gives verbal praise; repeats these trials a few times
Clinician	[*Re-presents the stimulus*] "Who are these?"	All cues faded; **an evoked trial**
Child	"Women."	A correct response
Clinician	"Excellent! You said *women*!"	Verbal praise; repeats evoked trials until the child gives 10 consecutively correct responses. Then teaches another baserated word.

Teach as many irregular plural words as you think are appropriate for the child. Use the following treatment recording sheet or print it from the CD.

Irregular Plural Words in Phrases
Exemplars and Treatment Recording Sheet

Print this page from the CD or photocopy this page for your clinical use.

Name/Age:	Date:
Goal: Production of the irregular plural words in phrases at 90% accuracy when asked questions and shown pictures.	Clinician:

Clinician's Comments:

Scoring: Correct: ✓   Incorrect or no response: X

Target skills	Discrete Trials														
	1	2	3	4	5	6	7	8	9	10	11	12	13	14	15
1. woman: two women															
2. man: two men															
3. child: three children															
4. foot: big feet															
5. tooth: many teeth															
6. goose: four geese															
7. mouse: three mice															
8. sheep: two sheep															

Teach 6 to 8 words each to a learning criterion of 10 consecutively correct, nonimitated (evoked) responses. Then, conduct a probe to assess generalized productions. Use the next page or print it from the CD.

Irregular Plural Words in Phrases

Probe Protocols and Recording Sheet

Print this page from the CD; the recording sheet on the CD shows several exemplars. You can also type in new exemplars.

Each time you teach 6 to 8 irregular plurals in phrases, conduct a probe to assess generalized production using varied pictures that represent the same target word. Find different pictures for the 6 to 8 trained plural nouns that have met the tentative training criterion of 10 consecutively correct responses on evoked trials. For instance, for the trained word women, select at least three (3) new pictures of women with different distinguishing features. Present each of these probe pictures of different women on a separate probe trial.

If the child fails to meet the probe criterion (90% correct) on untrained and varied representations of trained stimuli, give 4 to 6 training trials on each of the new probed stimuli. Then find additional and varied stimuli to readminister a probe. Alternate probes and treatment until the probe criterion is met.

Scripts for Probe Trials

Clinician	[Presents a new picture of *two women*] "Who are these?"	No modeling or prompts
Child	"Women." ["Two women."]	A correct probe response to a different picture of two women
Clinician	[Does not respond to the child's production]	No corrective feedback for any incorrect responses either

Name:	Date:	Session #:
Age:	**Clinician:**	
Disorder: Language	**Target Behavior: Irregular plural words in phrases**	
Untrained Stimuli	**Score: + correct; – incorrect or no responses**	
1a. pretty women (UT, new)		
1b. two women (UT, new)		
1c. five women (UT, new)		
2a. two men (UT, new)		
2b. three men (UT, new)		
2c. many men (UT, new)		
3a. three children (UT, new)		
3b. many children (UT, new)		
3c. some children (UT, new)		
4a. big feet (UT, new)		
4b. two feet (UT, new)		
4c. small feet (UT, new)		
Percent correct: (Criterion: 90%)		

UT = untrained, novel stimulus that may represent the same trained response (e.g., pictures of different-looking women or men than the ones used in teaching).

When the child meets the 90% correct probe criterion, select new irregular plurals for teaching. When you have taught a set of functional irregular plurals in phrases, teach them in sentences; follow the protocols on the next page.

Irregular Plural Words in Sentences
Treatment Protocols

Use the selected stimulus material to evoke speech in semicontrolled interactions.

Scripts for Modeled Sentence Production		Note
Clinician	[*Shows a large picture of a story scene in a story book*] "Who are these?" Say, **These are pretty women**."	Vocal emphasis on the target sentence
Child	"Pretty women."	Scored as a wrong response
Clinician	"Yes, but I want you to say the whole sentence, *These are pretty women*."	Corrective feedback
Clinician	[*Points to the target stimulus*] "Who are these? Say, **These are pretty women**."	Next trial
Child	"These are pretty women."	A correct response
Clinician	"Very good! You said *pretty women* in a sentence!"	Verbal praise

Repeat the trials until the child gives 5 consecutively correct, imitated responses. When the child imitates 5 correct modeled responses in sequence, fade the modeling. Each time, present the stimulus and point to it.

Scripts for More Spontaneous Conversation		Note
Clinician	[*Points to the target stimulus*] "These are pretty women. Who are these? Say, *these are . . .*"	Correct response modeled before the question
Child	"Pretty women"	A wrong response
Clinician	"Yes, but I want you to say the whole sentence, like you did before."	Corrective feedback
Clinician	"These are pretty women. Who are these? Say, *these are . . .*"	Next trial
Child	"These are pretty women."	A correct response; repeat these trials a few times
Clinician	"Very good! You said the whole sentence!"	Verbal praise
Clinician	"Who are these?"	All cues faded; **an evoked trial**
Child	"These are pretty women"	A correct response
Clinician	"Excellent! You said the whole sentence!"	Verbal praise
Clinician	"Now let us look at this picture here. What do you see here?"	A varied form of evoking a different irregular plural
Child	"I see many leaves."	A correct response
Clinician	"What color are the leaves? Start with the leaves are . . ."	Encouraging the use of the irregular plural in a different sentence
Child	"The leaf are green and brown"	A wrong response
Clinician	"They are green and brown. But remember to say *leaves*, not *leaf* when you see many like here."	Corrective feedback
Clinician	"What color are the leaves?"	Repeated trial
Child	"The leaves are green and brown."	Correct response; continues teaching in this manner

Irregular Plural Words in Sentences

Exemplars and Treatment Recording Sheet

Print this page from the CD or photocopy this page for your clinical use.

Name/Age:	Date:
Goal: Production of irregular plural words in sentences with 90% accuracy when asked questions while showing a picture or object.	Clinician:

Clinician's Comments:

Scoring: Correct: ✓ Incorrect or no response: X

Target skills	Discrete Trials														
	1	2	3	4	5	6	7	8	9	10	11	12	13	14	15
1. These are pretty women															
2. I see two men															
3. Here are three children															
4. They are big feet															
5. I see many teeth															
6. These are four geese															
7. I see three mice															
8. These are two sheep															

When the child has met the learning criterion of 10 consecutively correct, evoked (nonimitated) responses for each of the 6 to 8 target sentences, conduct a probe to see if the irregular plural word production has generalized to previously baserated but untrained sentences. Use the probe protocols given on the next page (or print it from the CD).

Irregular Plural Words in Sentences
Probe Protocols and Recording Sheet

Print this page from the CD; the recording sheet on the CD shows several exemplars. You can also type in new exemplars on the page shown in CD. **This page is for illustration only**.

Each time you teach 6 to 8 irregular plural sentences, conduct a probe to assess generalized production using varied pictures that represent the same target word. Find different pictures for the 6 to 8 trained plural nouns that have met the tentative training criterion of 10 consecutively correct responses on evoked trials. For instance, for the trained sentence these are pretty women, select at least three (3) new pictures of women with different distinguishing features. Present each of these probe pictures of different women on a separate probe trial.

Scripts for Probe Trials

Clinician:	[Presents a picture of *two new women*] "Who are these?"	No modeling or prompts
Child:	"These are women." ["These are pretty women."]	Correct probe responses to a different picture of two women
Clinician:	[Does not respond to the child's production]	No corrective feedback for any incorrect responses either

Name:	Date:	Session #:
Age:	**Clinician:**	
Disorder: Language	**Target Behavior: Irregular plural sentences**	
Trained and Untrained Stimuli	**Score: + correct; – incorrect or no responses**	
1a. These are pretty women (UT, new) 1b. Here are two women (UT, new) 1c. There are five women (UT, new)		
2a. I see two men (UT, new) 2b. Here are three men (UT, new) 2c. There are many men (UT, new)		
3a. Here are three children (UT, new) 3b. I see many children (UT, new) 3c. They are children (UT, new)		
4a. They are big feet (UT, new) 4b. I see two big feet (UT, new) 4c. These are big feet (UT, new)		
Percent correct probe (Criterion: 90%)		

UT = untrained, novel stimulus that may represent the same trained response (e.g., pictures of different-looking women or men than the ones used in teaching).

If the child fails to meet the probe criterion (90% correct) on untrained and varied representations of trained stimuli, give 4 to 6 training trials on each of the new probe stimuli. Then find additional and varied stimuli to readminister a probe. Alternate probes and treatment until the probe criterion is met.

When the child meets the probe criterion, select new irregular plurals for teaching. When you have taught a set of functional irregular plurals in sentences, move on to other morphologic features.

The Possessive Morphemes

Overview

Possession in English is expressed in varied forms. The most common bound possessive morpheme is a suffix and has three common allomorphic variations: the possessive s, z, and the ez. Each allomorphic variation is an independent response class as teaching one will not result in the automatic correct production of the other. For each allomorphic variation, only a few exemplars need to be taught to have the child produce the other exemplars on the basis of generalization. A possessive allomorph taught first (e.g., the s) may inappropriately generalize to words that take a different allomorph (e.g., the z). Therefore, the clinician needs to teach each of the variations.

The bound possessive morpheme is one of the early grammatic features children master. In Brown's (1973) study, the bound possessive was ranked number 6 to meet the acquisition criterion.

Other possessives are whole (free) morphemes. For instance, possessive also may be expressed with the irregular third person singular and plural forms *has* (e.g., *he has*, *she has*) and *have* (e.g., *they have*). In his study of morphologic learning in children, Brown (1973) tracked the irregular third person *has* and ranked it number 11 in meeting the mastery criterion.

Protocols are provided for possessive bound morphemes and free forms of irregular third person *has* and *have*.

General Training Strategy

The strategy to teach the possessive morpheme is similar to that used for the regular plural inflections. Each allomorphic variation may be baserated and taught in phrases and sentences. Some children may need to be taught the possessive at the word level to begin with. If so, the clinician may give a few trials on selected words with only the noun plus the possessive allomorph. When the initial level of training is words, the clinician may move to the sentence level without giving training at the phrase level. It is possible to move from the word level to the sentence level or initiate teaching at the phrase level with no word-level teaching. Experimentation with different starting points and skipped levels of training may result in more efficient teaching for many children.

The clinician should select 20 exemplars for each possessive allomorph, baserate them, teach them, periodically probe for generalized productions, and give additional training on those that do not result in generalized productions on probes.

Possessive *s*
Possessive *s* in Phrases
Baserate Protocols

On each trial, place a picture in front of the child to evoke the possessive s. Follow the protocol. Before asking the question, point to the thing possessed. Administer the evoked trials first followed by modeled trials. Do not provide feedback on any trials; just record the responses on the recording sheet provided on the next page or printed from the CD.

Scripts for Evoked Baserate Trial		Note
Clinician	[Pointing to the cat's bowl] "Whose bowl is this?	No modeling
Child	"Cat."	A wrong response
Clinician	Pulls the picture toward her and records the response.	No corrective feedback
Clinician	[Pointing to the giraffe's neck] "Whose neck is this?"	The next trial
Child	"Giraffe's."	A correct response
Clinician	Pulls the picture toward her and records the response.	No verbal praise

Administer the modeled baserate trials only after completing the evoked trials on all 20 (or more) exemplars. Again, place the relevant picture in front of the child before starting each trial.

Scripts for Modeled Baserate Trial		Note
Clinician	"This is the cat's bowl. Whose bowl is this? Say, *cat's bowl.*"	Modeling
Child	"Cat's bowl."	A wrong response
Clinician	Pulls the picture toward her and records the response.	No corrective feedback
Clinician	"This is the giraffe's neck. Whose neck is this? Say, the giraffe's neck."	Modeling
Child	"Giraffe's neck." ["The giraffe's neck."]	A correct response
Clinician	Pulls the picture toward her and records the response.	No verbal praise

Ignore the omission of the article.

Baserate at least 20 exemplars as shown on the next page.

Possessive *s* in Phrases

Exemplars and Baserate Recording Sheet

Print this page from the CD or photocopy this page for your clinical use.

Name/Age:	Date:
Goal: To establish the baserates of possessive *s* in phrases when asked questions while showing a picture or object.	Clinician:

Clinician's Comments:

Scoring: Correct: ✓   Incorrect or no response: X

Phrases with the Possessive *s*	Evoked	Modeled
1. Cat's bowl		
2. Giraffe's neck		
3. Sheep's hair		
4. Rabbit's tail		
5. Elephant's trunk		
6. Duck's feathers		
7. Bat's cave		
8. Nick's coat		
9. Rick's cap		
10. Goat's feet		
11. Rat's mouth		
12. Pat's bike		
13. Sheriff's badge		
14. Beth's bag		
15. Mike's ball.		
16. Matt's chair		
17. Chuck's hat		
18. Kate's ring		
19. Jack's pencil		
20. Snake's tongue		
Percent correct baserate		

Replace or add exemplars as you see fit for the child.

After establishing the baserates of possessive s *in phrases, begin teaching them. Use the protocols given on the next page.*

Possessive *s* in Phrases

Treatment Protocols

At the beginning of each trial, place a picture in front of the child (e.g., one showing a cat and a bowl). At the beginning of each trial, point to the person and the object.

Scripts for Modeled Discrete Trial Training		Note
Clinician	"This is the cat's bowl. Whose bowl is this? Say, *the cat's bowl.*"	Vocal emphasis on the target morpheme
Client	"Cat bowl."	A wrong response
Clinician	"No, that is not correct. Whose bowl is this? Say, *the cat's bowl.*"	Corrective feedback; vocal emphasis on the possessive
Client	"Cat's bowl."	A correct response
Clinician	"Very good! You said *cat's*, not *cat!*"	Verbal praise

Repeat the trials until the child gives 5 consecutively correct, imitated responses. When the child imitates 5 correct responses in sequence, fade the modeling. Each time, point to the correct stimulus. Always show a picture before asking a question.

Scripts for Fading the Modeling		Note
Clinician	"This is the cat's bowl. Whose bowl is this? Say, cat . . ."	Partial modeling only
Client	"Cat bowl."	A wrong response
Clinician	"No, that is not correct; don't forget the *s*. Whose bowl is this? Say, *cat . . .*"	Corrective feedback and partial modeling
Client	"Cat's bowl."	A correct response
Clinician	"Very good! You said *cat's*, not *cat!*"	Verbal praise
Clinician	"This is the cat's bowl. Whose bowl is this?"	Reduced cues; no prompts
Client	"Cat's bowl." ["The cat's bowl"]	Both the forms accepted
Clinician	"Excellent! You said *cat's bowl!*"	Verbal praise
Clinician	"Whose bowl is this?"	**An Evoked Trial**
Client	"Cat's bowl."	Typically correct answer

If the wrong responses persist on 4 to 5 evoked trials, reinstate partial or full modeling for a few trials, again fade the modeling, and re-present the evoked trials.

When the child meets the tentative learning criterion of 10 consecutively correct, nonimitated responses for a given stimulus item, move on to the next stimulus item. With this procedure, teach 6 to 8 exemplars using the recording sheet shown on the following page. Use different exemplars as you see fit for a given child. Print the recording sheet from the CD or photocopy the next page for your clinical use.

Possessive *s* in Phrases

Exemplars and Treatment Recording Sheet

Print this page from the CD or photocopy this page for your clinical use.

Teach 6 to 8 exemplars using the previous scripts.

Name/Age:	Date:
Goal: Production of the possessive *s* in phrases with 90% accuracy.	Clinician:

Clinician's Comments:

Scoring: Correct: ✓   Incorrect or no response: X

Target skills	Discrete Trials														
	1	2	3	4	5	6	7	8	9	10	11	12	13	14	15
1. Kitty's bowl															
2. Giraffe's neck															
3. Sheep's hair															
4. Rabbit's tail															
5. Elephant's trunk															
6. Duck's feathers															
7. Bat's cave															
8. Nick's coat															

Teach 6 to 8 exemplars each to a training criterion of 10 consecutively correct, nonimitated responses. Then, teach the possessive s *in sentences; probes may be unnecessary at the phrase level.*

Possessive *s* in Sentences

Baserate Protocols

At the beginning of each trial, place a relevant picture in front of the child. Point to the noun and the object being possessed and then ask the specified question. Do not respond in any way to the child's correct, incorrect, or lack of response.

Scripts for Evoked Baserate Trial		Note
Clinician	"Whose bowl is this?"	No modeling; evoked trial
Child	"Cat's." ["Kitty's bowl]	A wrong response
Clinician	Pulls the picture toward her and records the response.	No corrective feedback
Clinician	"Whose neck is it? Start with *it is the . . .*"	Prompts the sentence
Child	"It is the giraffe's neck."	A correct response
Clinician	Pulls the picture toward her and records the response.	No verbal praise

Administer the modeled baserate trials only after completing the evoked trials on all 20 (or more) exemplars. Again, place a relevant picture in front of the child at the beginning of each trial and then ask the question.

Scripts for Modeled Baserate Trial		Note
Clinician	"Whose bowl is this? Say, *it is the cat's bowl.*"	Modeled trial
Child	"It is cat's bowl."	A wrong response
Clinician	Pulls the picture toward her and records the response.	No corrective feedback
Clinician	"Whose neck is it? Say, *it is the giraffe's neck.*"	Another modeled trial
Child	"It is the giraffe's neck."	A correct response
Clinician	Pulls the picture toward her and records the response.	No verbal praise

Use the exemplars and the recording sheet given on the next page to establish the baserates of the possessive s *in sentences (or print it from the CD).*

Possessive *s* in Sentences

Exemplars and Baserate Recording Sheet

Print this page from the CD or photocopy this page for your clinical use.

Name/Age:	Date:
Goal: To establish the baserates of the possessive *s* in sentences when asked questions while showing a picture or object.	Clinician:

Clinician's Comments:

Scoring: Correct: ✓ Incorrect or no response: X

Sentence Level	Evoked	Modeled
1. It is the cat's bowl.		
2. It is the giraffe's neck.		
3. It is the sheep's hair.		
4. It is the rabbit's tail.		
5. It is the elephant's trunk.		
6. It is the duck's feathers.		
7. It is the bat's cave.		
8. It is Nick's coat.		
9. It is Rick's cap.		
10. It is the goat's head.		
11. It is the rat's mouth.		
12. It is Pat's bike.		
13. It is the sheriff's badge.		
14. It is Beth's bag.		
15. It is Mike's ball.		
16. It is Matt's chair.		
17. It is Chuck's hat.		
18. It is Kate's ring.		
19. It is Jack's pencil.		
20. It is snake's tongue.		
Percent correct baserate		

Replace or add new exemplars as you see fit for a given child.

After establishing the baserates for the possessive s *in sentences, initiate treatment. Use the protocols given on the next page.*

Possessive *s* in Sentences

Treatment Protocols

Teach 6 to 8 sentences with the possessive s using the following script.

Place a picture in front of the child that shows a noun and an object being possessed. At the beginning of each trial, point to the noun and the object.

Scripts for Modeled Discrete Trial Training		Note
Clinician	"It is the cat's bowl. Whose bowl is it? Say, *it is the cat's bowl.*"	Modeling; the target vocally emphasized
Child	"Cat bowl."	A wrong response
Clinician	"No, that's not correct. You forgot the **s** sound. ["No, you didn't say the whole sentence."]	Corrective feedback; the trial scored as incorrect
Clinician	"It is the cat's bowl. Whose bowl is this? Say, *It is the cat's bowl.*"	The next trial
Child	"It is the cat's bowl."	A correct response
Clinician	"Excellent! You said the whole sentence correctly!"	Verbal praise

Repeat the trials until the child gives 5 consecutively correct, imitated responses. When the child imitates 5 correct responses in sequence, fade the modeling. Each time, present and point to the correct stimulus.

Scripts for Fading the Modeling		Note
Clinician	"Whose bowl is it? Say, *it is the . . .*"	Partial modeling only
Child	"Cat's."	Scored as a wrong response
Clinician	"No, that is not correct. You didn't say all of it."	Corrective feedback; scored as incorrect
Clinician	"Whose bowl is it? Say, *it is the . . .*"	The next trial
Child	"It is the cat's bowl."	A correct response
Clinician	"Excellent! You said the whole sentence!"	Verbal praise
Clinician	"Whose bowl is it?"	Typical question; **an evoked trial**
Child	"It is the cat's bowl."	A correct response

If the wrong responses persist on 4 to 5 evoked trials, reinstate partial or full modeling for a few trials, again fade the modeling, and re-present the evoked trials.

When the child meets the tentative learning criterion of 10 consecutively correct, nonimitated responses for a given stimulus item, move on to the next stimulus item. With this procedure, teach 6 to 8 exemplars shown on the following recording sheet. Use different exemplars as you see fit for a given child.

Possessive *s* in Sentences

Exemplars and Treatment Recording Sheet

Print this page from the CD or photocopy this page for your clinical use.

Name/Age:	Date:
Goal: Production of the possessive *s* in sentences with 90% accuracy when asked questions while showing a picture or object.	Clinician:

Clinician's Comments:

Scoring: Correct: ✓   Incorrect or no response: X

Target skills	Discrete Trials														
	1	2	3	4	5	6	7	8	9	10	11	12	13	14	15
1. It is the cat's bowl.															
2. It is the giraffe's neck.															
3. It is the sheep's hair.															
4. It is the rabbit's tail.															
5. It is the elephant's trunk.															
6. It is the duck's feathers.															
7. It is Nick's coat.															
8. It is the girl's coat.															

When the child has met the learning criterion of 10 consecutively correct, evoked (nonimitated) responses for each of the 6 to 8 target sentences, conduct a probe to see if the possessive s production has generalized to previously baserated but untrained sentences.

Use the probe protocol given on the next page.

Possessive *s* in Sentences

Probe Protocols and Recording Sheet

Print this page from the CD or photocopy this page for your clinical use.

On the probes, present only the untrained exemplars (UT). When the child fails to meet the 90% correct probe criterion, either teach 2 to 4 new exemplars or give additional training trials on already trained stimuli. If needed, select new exemplars for probes. Probe at least 10 untrained exemplars. Alternate probes and treatment until the probe criterion is met.

Scripts for Probe Trials

Clinician	[Presents an untrained stimulus] "Whose cap is it?"	No modeling or prompts
Child	"It is Rick's cap."	A correct, generalized response
Clinician	Scores the response as correct.	Offers no reinforcement
Clinician	[Presents another untrained stimulus] "Whose head is it?"	The second probe trial
Child	"Goat head."	A wrong probe response
Clinician	Scores the response as incorrect.	Offers no corrective feedback

Name:		Date:	Session #:
Age:		Clinician:	
Disorder: Language		Target: Possessive *s* in sentences (probe)	
Untrained Stimuli		**Score: + correct; – incorrect or no responses**	
1. It is Rick's cap.			
2. It is the goat's head.			
3. It is the rat's mouth.			
4. It is Pat's bike.			
5. It is the sheriff's badge.			
6. It is Beth's bag.			
7. It is Mike's ball.			
8. It is Matt's chair.			
9. It is Chuck's hat.			
10. It is Kate's ring.			
11. It is Jack's pencil.			
12. It is the snake's tongue.			
Percent correct probe (Criterion: 90%)			

If the child does not meet the probe criterion, give additional training on already trained sentences and subsequently, readminister the probe trials. When the child meets the 90% correct probe criterion for the possessive s in sentences, shift training to other morphologic features or to conversational speech in which the possessive s is monitored and reinforced.

Possessive z
Possessive z in Phrases
Baserate Protocols

Possessive z is an allomorphic variation of the possessive morpheme. Although spelled with an s, it is pronounced as z when the noun with which it is suffixed ends with a voiced phoneme (e.g., as in *King's*). Children who are taught one of the allomorphic variations of the possessive may inappropriately generalize its production to contexts in which a different allomorphic variation needs to be used. Therefore, the possessive z is a separate treatment target for children with language disorders.

On each trial, place a picture in front of the child to evoke the possessive z. Follow the protocol. Before asking the question, point to the thing possessed. Administer the evoked trials first followed by modeled trials. Do not provide feedback on any trials; just record the responses on the recording sheet provided on the next page or printed from the CD.

Scripts for Evoked Baserate Trial		Note
Clinician	[Pointing to the baby's bottle] "Whose bottle is this?	No modeling
Child	"Baby."	A wrong response
Clinician	Pulls the picture toward her and records the response.	No corrective feedback
Clinician	[Pointing to the bear's cave] "Whose cave is this?"	The next trial
Child	"Bear's."	A correct response
Clinician	Pulls the picture toward her and records the response.	No verbal praise

Administer the modeled baserate trials only after completing the evoked trials on all 20 (or more) exemplars. Again, place the relevant picture in front of the child before starting each trial.

Scripts for Modeled Baserate Trial		Note
Clinician	"This is the baby's bottle. Whose bottle is this? Say, *baby's bottle*."	Modeling
Child	"Baby's bottle."	A correct response
Clinician	Pulls the picture toward her and records the response.	No verbal praise
Clinician	"This is the bear's cave. Whose cave is this? Say, *the bear's cave*."	Modeling
Child	"Bear's cave." ["The bear's cave."]	A correct response
Clinician	Pulls the picture toward her and records the response.	No verbal praise

Ignore the omission of the article.

Baserate at least 20 exemplars as shown on the next page.

Possessive z in Phrases

Exemplars and Baserate Recording Sheet

Print this page from the CD or photocopy this page for your clinical use.

Name/Age:	Date:
Goal: To establish the baserates of the possessive z in phrases when asked questions while showing a picture or object.	Clinician:

Clinician's Comments:

Scoring: Correct: ✓   Incorrect or no response: X

Phrases with the Possessive z	Evoked	Modeled
1. the baby's bottle.		
2. the bear's cave.		
3. the bird's nest.		
4. the boy's balloon.		
5. daddy's car.		
6. Jan's house.		
7. the farmer's tractor.		
8. the girl's bike.		
9. the doctor's office.		
10. the king's army.		
11. the woman's purse.		
12. the lion's mouth.		
13. the man's hat.		
14. the Mommy's key.		
15. the monkey's banana.		
16. the painter's brush.		
17. the pig's tail.		
18. the queen's crown.		
19. the captain's ship.		
20. the teacher's apple.		
Percent correct baserate		

Replace or add exemplars as you see fit for the child.

After establishing the baserates of possessive z in phrases, begin teaching them. Use the protocols given on the next page.

Possessive *z* in Phrases

Treatment Protocols

At the beginning of each trial, place a picture in front of the child (e.g., one showing a cat and a bowl). At the beginning of each trial, point to the person and the object.

Scripts for Modeled Discrete Trial Training		Note
Clinician	"This is the baby's bottle. Whose bottle is this? Say, *the baby's bottle.*"	Vocal emphasis on the target morpheme
Client	"Baby bottle."	A wrong response
Clinician	"No, that is not correct. What are these? Say, *the baby's bottle.*"	Corrective feedback; vocal emphasis on the possessive
Client	"Baby's bottle."	A correct response
Clinician	"Very good! You said *baby's*, not *baby*!"	Verbal praise

Repeat the trials until the child gives 5 consecutively correct, imitated responses. When the child imitates 5 correct responses in sequence, fade the modeling. Each time, point to the correct stimulus. Always show a picture before asking a question.

Scripts for Fading the Modeling		Note
Clinician	"This is the baby's bottle. Whose bottle is this? Say, baby . . ."	Partial modeling only
Client	"Baby bottle."	A wrong response
Clinician	"No, that is not correct; don't forget the z. Whose bottle is this? Say, *baby* . . ."	Corrective feedback and partial modeling
Client	"Baby's bottle."	A correct response
Clinician	"Very good! You said *baby's*, not *baby*!"	Verbal praise
Clinician	"This is the baby's bottle. Whose bottle is this?"	Reduced cues; no prompts
Client	"Baby's bottle." ["The baby's bottle."]	Both the forms accepted
Clinician	"Excellent! You said *baby's bottle*!"	Verbal praise
Clinician	"Whose bottle is this?"	**An Evoked Trial**
Client	"Baby's bottle." ["The baby's bottle."]	Typically correct answer

If the wrong responses persist on 4 to 5 evoked trials, reinstate partial or full modeling for a few trials, again fade the modeling, and re-present the evoked trials.

When the child meets the tentative learning criterion of 10 consecutively correct, nonimitated responses for a given stimulus item, move on to the next stimulus item. With this procedure, teach 6 to 8 exemplars using the recording sheet shown on the following page. Use different exemplars as you see fit for a given child. Print the recording sheet from the CD or photocopy the next page for your clinical use.

Possessive *z* in Phrases

Exemplars and Treatment Recording Sheet

Print this page from the CD or photocopy this page for your clinical use.

Teach 6 to 8 exemplars using the previous scripts.

Name/Age:	Date:
Goal: Production of the possessive *z* in phrases with 90% accuracy when asked questions while showing pictures or objects.	Clinician:

Clinician's Comments:

Scoring: Correct: ✓   Incorrect or no response: X

Target skills	Discrete Trials														
	1	2	3	4	5	6	7	8	9	10	11	12	13	14	15
1. The baby's bottle															
2. The bear's cave															
3. The bird's nest															
4. The boy's balloon															
5. Daddy's car															
6. Man's house															
7. The farmer's tractor															
8. Girl's bike															

Teach 8 to 10 exemplars each to a training criterion of 10 consecutively correct, nonimitated responses. Then, move on to training the production of the possessive z in sentences

Possessive z in Sentences

Baserate Protocols

At the beginning of each trial, place a relevant picture in front of the child. Point to the noun and the object being possessed and then ask the specified question. Do not respond in any way to the child's correct, incorrect, or lack of responses.

Scripts for Evoked Baserate Trial		Note
Clinician	"Whose bottle is this? Start with, *this is . . .*"	Prompting the longer sentence form
Child	"Baby's." ["Baby's bottle."]	A wrong response
Clinician	Pulls the picture toward her and records the response.	No corrective feedback
Clinician	"Whose cave is this? Start with, *this is . . .*"	Prompts the sentence
Child	"This is the bear's cave."	A correct response
Clinician	Pulls the picture toward her and records the response.	No verbal praise

Administer the modeled baserate trials only after completing the evoked trials on all 20 (or more) exemplars. Again, place a relevant picture in front of the child at the beginning of each trial and then ask the question.

Scripts for Modeled Baserate Trial		Note
Clinician	"Whose bottle is this? Say, *this is the baby's bottle.*"	Modeled trial
Child	"Baby's bottle."	A wrong response
Clinician	Pulls the picture toward her and records the response.	No corrective feedback
Clinician	"Whose cave is this? Say, *this is the bear's cave.*"	Another modeled trial
Child	"This is the bear's cave."	A correct response
Clinician	Pulls the picture toward her and records the response.	No verbal praise

Use the exemplars and the recording sheet given on the next page to establish the baserates of the possessive z in sentences (or print it from the CD).

Possessive z in Sentences

Exemplars and Baserate Recording Sheet

Print this page from the CD or photocopy this page for your clinical use.

Name/Age:	Date:
Goal: To establish the baserates of possessive z in sentences when asked questions while showing a picture or object.	Clinician:

Clinician's Comments:

Scoring: Correct: ✓ Incorrect or no response: X

Sentence Level	Evoked	Modeled
1. This is the baby's bottle.		
2. This is the bear's cave.		
3. This is the bird's nest.		
4. This is the boy's balloon.		
5. This is Daddy's car.		
6. This is the doctor's office.		
7. This is the farmer's animals.		
8. This is the girl's bike.		
9. This is Jan's house.		
10. This is the king's army.		
11. This is the woman's purse.		
12. This is the lion's mouth.		
13. This is the man's hat.		
14. This is the Mommy's key.		
15. This is the monkey's banana.		
16. This is the painter's brush.		
17. This is the pig's tail.		
18. This is the queen's crown.		
19. This is the captain's ship.		
20. This is the teacher's apple.		
Percent correct baserate		

Replace or add new exemplars as you see fit for a given child.

After establishing the baserates for the possessive z in sentences, initiate treatment. Use the protocols given on the next page.

Possessive z in Sentences

Treatment Protocols

Teach 6 to 8 sentences with the plural z using the following script.

Place a picture in front of the child that shows a noun and an object being possessed. At the beginning of each trial, point to the noun and the object.

Scripts for Modeled Discrete Trial Training		Note
Clinician	"This is the baby's bottle. Whose bottle is this? Say, *this is the baby's bottle.*"	Modeling; the target vocally emphasized
Child	"Baby bottle."	A wrong response
Clinician	"No, that's not correct. You forgot the **z** sound. ["No, you didn't say the whole sentence."]	Corrective feedback; the trial scored as incorrect
Clinician	This is the baby's bottle. Whose bottle is this? Say, *This is the baby's bottle.*"	The next trial
Child	"This is the baby's bottle."	A correct response
Clinician	"Excellent! You said the whole sentence correctly!"	Verbal praise

Repeat the trials until the child gives 5 consecutively correct, imitated responses. When the child imitates 5 correct responses in sequence, fade the modeling. Each time, present and point to the correct stimulus.

Scripts for Fading the Modeling		Note
Clinician	"Whose bottle is this? Say, *this is the . . .* "	Partial modeling only
Child	"Baby's."	Scored as a wrong response
Clinician	"No, that is not correct. You didn't say all of it."	Corrective feedback; scored as incorrect
Clinician	Whose bottle is this? Say, *this is the . . .* "	The next trial
Child	"This is the baby's bottle."	A correct response
Clinician	"Excellent! You said the whole sentence!"	Verbal praise
Clinician	"Whose bottle is this?"	Typical question; **an evoked trial**
Child	"This is the baby's bottle."	A correct response

If the wrong responses persist on 4 to 5 evoked trials, reinstate partial or full modeling for a few trials, again fade the modeling, and re-present the evoked trials.

When the child meets the tentative learning criterion of 10 consecutively correct, nonimitated responses for a given stimulus item, move on to the next stimulus item. With this procedure, teach 6 to 8 exemplars shown on the following recording sheet. Use different exemplars as you see fit for a given child.

Possessive z in Sentences

Exemplars and Treatment Recording Sheet

Print this page from the CD or photocopy this page for your clinical use.

Name/Age:	Date:
Goal: Production of the possessive z in sentences with 90% accuracy when asked questions while showing pictures or objects.	Clinician:

Clinician's Comments:

Scoring: Correct: ✓   Incorrect or no response: X

Target skills	Discrete Trials														
	1	2	3	4	5	6	7	8	9	10	11	12	13	14	15
1. This is the baby's bottle.															
2. This is the bear's cave.															
3. This is the bird's nest.															
4. This is the boy's balloon.															
5. This is Daddy's car.															
6. This is the doctor's office.															
7. This is the farmer's animals.															
8. This is the girl's bike.															

When the child has met the learning criterion of 10 consecutively correct evoked (nonimitated) responses for each of the 6 to 8 target sentences, conduct a probe to see if the possessive z production has generalized to previously baserated but untrained sentences.

Use the protocol given on the next page.

Possessive *z* in Sentences

Probe Protocols and Recording Sheet

Print this page from the CD or photocopy this page for your clinical use.

On the probes, present only the untrained exemplars (UT). When the child fails to meet the 90% correct probe criterion, either teach 2 to 4 new exemplars or give additional training trials on already trained stimuli. If needed, select new exemplars for probes. Probe at least 10 untrained exemplars. Alternate probes and treatment until the probe criterion is met.

Scripts for Probe Trials

Clinician	[Presents an untrained stimulus] "Whose house is it?"	No modeling or prompts
Child	"It is Jan's house."	A correct, generalized response
Clinician	Scores the response as correct.	Offers no reinforcement
Clinician	[Presents another untrained stimulus] "Whose army is it?"	The second probe trial
Child	"King."	A wrong probe response
Clinician	Scores the response as incorrect.	Offers no corrective feedback

Name:	Date:	Session #:
Age:	**Clinician:**	
Disorder: Language	**Target: Possessive *z* in sentences (probe)**	
Untrained Stimuli	**Score: + correct; – incorrect or no responses**	
1. This is Jan's house.		
2. This is the king's army.		
3. This is the woman's purse.		
4. This is the lion's mouth.		
5. This is the man's hat.		
6. This is the Mommy's key.		
7. This is the monkey's banana.		
8. This is the painter's brush.		
9. This is the pig's tail.		
10. This is the queen's crown.		
11. This is the captain's ship.		
12. This is the teacher's apple.		
Percent correct probe (Criterion: 90%)		

If the child does not meet the probe criterion, give additional training on already trained sentences and subsequently readminister the probe trials. When the child meets the 90% correct probe criterion for the possessive z in sentences, shift training to other morphologic features or to conversational speech in which the possessive z is monitored and reinforced.

Possessive *ez*
Possessive *ez* in Words or Phrases
Baserate Protocols

Possessive *ez* is an allomorphic variation of the possessive morpheme. Variously spelled *e's* (e.g., *judge's*), *s's* (e.g., *Lewis's*), or *ss's* (*waitress's*), the allomorph is pronounced as z. Children who are taught one of the allomorphic variations of the possessive may inappropriately generalize its production to contexts in which a different allomorphic variation needs to be used. Therefore, the possessive *ez* is a separate treatment target for children with language disorders.

On each trial, place a picture in front of the child to evoke the possessive ez. Follow the protocol. Before asking the question, point to the thing possessed. Administer the evoked trials first followed by modeled trials. Do not provide feedback on any trials; just record the child's responses on the recording sheet provided on the next page or printed from the CD.

Although the protocols and the subsequent exemplars show complete sentences, score the response as correct if the child produced the possessive ez in at least the word. Ignore the omission of the initial articles.

Scripts for Evoked Baserate Trial		Note
Clinician	[Pointing to the horse's tail] "Whose tail is long?"	No modeling
Child	"Horse."	A wrong response
Clinician	Pulls the picture toward her and records the response.	No corrective feedback
Clinician	[Pointing to the judge's gown] "Whose gown is black?"	The next trial; if the child did not know the word *judge*, say, "this is a judge, wearing a black gown. Whose gown is black?"
Child	"Judge's."	A correct response
Clinician	Pulls the picture toward her and records the response.	No verbal praise

Administer the modeled baserate trials only after completing the evoked trials on all 15 (or more) exemplars. Again, place the relevant picture in front of the child before starting each trial.

Scripts for Modeled Baserate Trial		Note
Clinician	"This is the horse's long tail. Whose tail is long? Say, *the horse's.*"	Modeling
Child	"Horse." ["The horse."]	A wrong response
Clinician	Pulls the picture toward her and records the response.	No corrective feedback
Clinician	"This is the judge's black gown. Whose gown is black? Say, *the judge's.*"	Modeling
Child	"Judge's." ["The judge's."]	A correct response
Clinician	Pulls the picture toward her and records the response.	No verbal praise

Ignore the omission of the article.

Baserate at least 15 stimulus pictures as shown on the next page (ez is a relatively uncommon possessive allomorph and it is difficult to find functional ez possessive nouns in large numbers).

Possessive *ez* in Words or Phrases

Exemplars and Baserate Recording Sheet

Print this page from the CD or photocopy this page for your clinical use.

Name/Age:	Date:
Goal: To establish the baserates of possessive *ez* in phrases when asked questions while showing a picture or object.	Clinician:

Clinician's Comments:

Scoring: Correct: ✓   Incorrect or no response: X

Phrases with the Possessive *ez*	Evoked	Modeled
1. The horse's [tail is long.]		
2. The judge's [gown is black.]		
3. The mouse's [home is small.]		
4. The nurse's [uniform is white.]		
5. The police's [car is blue.]		
6. Santa Claus's [elves are strong.]		
7. The tortoise's [shell is green.]		
8. The waitress' s [table is red.]		
9. The walrus' s [cage is big.]		
10. The witch's [broom is old.]		
11. Bryce's [hat is yellow.]		
12. The moose's [antlers are sharp.]		
13. Denise's [pen is purple.]		
14. Janice's [mittens are warm.]		
15. Louise's [dog is jumping.]		
16. The stewardess's dress is nice.		
17. The goose's feathers are white.		
Percent correct baserate		

Replace or add exemplars as you see fit for the child.

After establishing the baserates of possessive ez in words or phrases, begin teaching them. Use the protocols given on the next page.

Possessive *ez* in Words or Phrases

Treatment Protocols

At the beginning of each trial, place a picture in front of the child, point to the noun and the object being possessed.

Scripts for Modeled Discrete Trial Training		Note
Clinician	"This is the horse's long tail. Whose tail is long? Say, *the horse's tail*."	Vocal emphasis on the target morpheme
Client	"Horse tail." ["The horse tail."]	A wrong response
Clinician	"No, that is not correct. Whose tail is long? Say, *the horse's tail*."	Corrective feedback; vocal emphasis on the possessive
Client	"Horse's tail." ["The horse's tail."]	A correct response
Clinician	"Very good! You said *horse's*, not *horse!*"	Verbal praise

Repeat the trials until the child gives 5 consecutively correct, imitated responses. When the child imitates 5 correct responses in sequence, fade the modeling. Each time, point to the correct stimulus. Always show a picture before asking a question.

Scripts for Fading the Modeling		Note
Clinician	"This is the horse's long tail. Whose tail long? Say, the horse . . . "	Partial modeling only
Client	"Horse tail."	A wrong response
Clinician	"No, that is not correct; don't forget the *ez*. Whose tail is long? Say, *the horse* . . . "	Corrective feedback and partial modeling
Client	"horse's tail."	A correct response
Clinician	"Very good! You said *horse's*, not *horse!*"	Verbal praise
Clinician	"This is the horse's long tail. Whose tail is this?"	Reduced cues; no prompts
Client	"Horse's tail." ["The horse's tail"]	Both the forms accepted
Clinician	"Excellent! You said *horse's tail!*"	Verbal praise
Clinician	"Whose long tail is this?"	**An Evoked Trial**
Client	"The horse's tail."	Typically correct answer

If the wrong responses persist on 4 to 5 evoked trials, reinstate partial or full modeling for a few trials, again fade the modeling, and re-present the evoked trials.

When the child meets the tentative learning criterion of 10 consecutively correct, nonimitated responses for a given stimulus item, move on to the next stimulus item. With this procedure, teach 6 to 8 exemplars using the recording sheet shown on the following page. Use different exemplars as you see fit for a given child. Print the recording sheet from the CD or photocopy the next page for your clinical use.

Possessive *ez* in Words or Phrases

Exemplars and Treatment Recording Sheet

Print this page from the CD or photocopy this page for your clinical use.

Teach 6 to 8 exemplars using the previous scripts.

Name/Age:	Date:
Goal: Production of the possessive *ez* in words or phrases with 90% accuracy when asked questions while showing pictures.	Clinician:

Clinician's Comments:

Scoring: Correct: ✓ Incorrect or no response: X

Target skills	Discrete Trials														
	1	2	3	4	5	6	7	8	9	10	11	12	13	14	15
1. The horse's [tail is long.]															
2. The judge's [gown is black.]															
3. The mouse's [home is small.]															
4. The nurse's [uniform is white.]															
5. The police's [car is blue.]															
6. Santa Claus's [elves are strong.]															
7. The tortoise's [shell is green.]															
8. The waitress's [table is red.]															
9. The walrus's [cage is big.]															
10. The witch's [broom is old.]															

Teach 8 to 10 exemplars each to a training criterion of 10 consecutively correct, nonimitated responses. Then, move on to baserating and teaching the production of the possessive ez in sentences

Possessive *ez* in Sentences

Baserate Protocols

At the beginning of each trial, place a relevant picture in front of the child. Point to the noun and what is being possessed and then ask the specified question. Do not respond in any way to the child's correct, incorrect, or lack of response.

Scripts for Evoked Baserate Trial		Note
Clinician	[Pointing to the horse's tail] "Whose tail is long?"	No modeling; evoked trial
Child	"Horse's." ["The horse's tail."]	A wrong response
Clinician	Pulls the picture toward her and records the response.	No corrective feedback
Clinician	[Pointing to the judge's gown] "Whose gown is black? Start with *the judge* . . ."	Prompts the sentence
Child	"The judge's gown is black."	A correct response
Clinician	Pulls the picture toward her and records the response.	No verbal praise

Administer the modeled baserate trials only after completing the evoked trials on all 20 (or more) exemplars. Again, place a relevant picture in front of the child at the beginning of each trial and then ask the question.

Scripts for Modeled Baserate Trial		Note
Clinician	"Whose tail is long?"? Say, *the horse's tail is long.*"	Modeled trial
Child	"Horse's tail."	A wrong response
Clinician	Pulls the picture toward her and records the response.	No corrective feedback
Clinician	"Whose gown is black? Say, *the judge's gown is black.*"	Another modeled trial
Child	"The judge's gown is black."	A correct response
Clinician	Pulls the picture toward her and records the response.	No verbal praise

Use the exemplars and the recording sheet given on the next page (or print it from the CD) to establish the baserates of the possessive ez in sentences.

Possessive *ez* in Sentences

Exemplars and Baserate Recording Sheet

Print this page from CD or photocopy this page for your clinical use.

Name/Age:	Date:
Goal: To establish the baserates of possessive *ez* in sentences when asked questions while showing a picture or object.	Clinician:

Clinician's Comments:

Scoring: Correct: ✓   Incorrect or no response: X

Sentence Level	Evoked	Modeled
1. The horse's tail is long.		
2. The judge's gown is black.		
3. The mouse's home is small.		
4. The nurse's uniform is white.		
5. The police's car is blue.		
6. Santa Claus's elves are strong.		
7. The tortoise's shell is green.		
8. The waitress' s table is red.		
9. The walrus' s cage is big.		
10. The witch's broom is old.		
11. Bryce's hat is yellow.		
12. The moose's antlers are sharp.		
13. Denise's pen is purple.		
14. Janice's mittens are warm.		
15. Louise's dog is jumping.		
16. The stewardess's dress is nice.		
17. The goose's feathers are white.		
Percent correct baserate		

Replace or add new exemplars as you see fit for a given child.

After establishing the baserates for the possessive ez in sentences, initiate treatment. Use the protocols given on the next page.

Possessive *ez* in Sentences

Treatment Protocols

Teach 8 to 10 sentences with the possessive ez using the following script.

Place a picture in front of the child that shows a noun and what is possessed. At the beginning of each trial, point to the noun and the possession.

Scripts for Modeled Discrete Trial Training		Note
Clinician	"The horse's tail is long. Whose tail is long? Say, *the horse's tail is long.*"	Modeling; the target vocally emphasized
Child	"Horse tail."	A wrong response
Clinician	"No, that's not correct. you forgot the **ez** sound. ["No, you didn't say the whole sentence."]	Corrective feedback; the trial scored as incorrect
Clinician	"The horse's tail is long. Whose tail is long? Say, *the horse's tail is long.*"	The next trial
Child	"The horse's tail is long." ["Horse's tail is long."]	A correct response
Clinician	"Excellent! You said the whole sentence correctly!"	Verbal praise

Repeat the trials until the child gives 5 consecutively correct, imitated responses. When the child imitates 5 correct responses in sequence, fade the modeling. Each time, present and point to the correct stimulus elements.

Scripts for Fading the Modeling		Note
Clinician	"Whose tail is long? Say, *the horse . . .*"	Partial modeling only
Child	"Horse's."	Scored as a wrong response
Clinician	"No, that is not correct. You didn't say all of it."	Corrective feedback; scored as incorrect
Clinician	Whose tail is long? Say, *the horse . . .*"	The next trial
Child	"The horse's tail is long."	A correct response
Clinician	"Excellent! You said the whole sentence!"	Verbal praise
Clinician	"Whose tail is long?"	Typical question; **an evoked trial**
Child	"The horse's tail is long."	A correct response
Clinician	"Excellent! You said the whole sentence!"	Verbal praise

If the wrong responses persist on 4 to 5 evoked trials, reinstate partial or full modeling for a few trials, again fade the modeling, and re-present the evoked trials.

When the child meets the tentative learning criterion of 10 consecutively correct, nonimitated responses for a given stimulus item, move on to the next stimulus item. With this procedure, teach 6 to 8 exemplars shown on the following recording sheet. Use different exemplars as you see fit for a given child.

Possessive *ez* in Sentences

Exemplars and Treatment Recording Sheet

Print this page from the CD or photocopy this page for your clinical use.

Name/Age:	Date:
Goal: Production of the possessive *ez* in sentences with 90% accuracy when asked questions while showing pictures.	Clinician:

Clinician's Comments:

Scoring: Correct: ✓   Incorrect or no response: X

Target skills	Discrete Trials														
	1	2	3	4	5	6	7	8	9	10	11	12	13	14	15
1. The horse's tail is long.															
2. The judge's gown is black.															
3. The mouse's home is small.															
4. The nurse's uniform is white.															
5. The police's car is blue.															
6. Santa Claus's elves are strong.															
7. The tortoise's shell is green.															
8. The waitress's table is red.															
9. The walrus's cage is big.															
10. The witch's broom is old.															

When the child has met the learning criterion of 10 consecutively correct, evoked (nonimitated) responses for each of the 8 to 10 target sentences, conduct a probe to see if the possessive ez production has generalized to untrained sentences. Use the protocols given on the next page.

Possessive *ez* in Sentences
Probe Protocols and Recording Sheet

Print this page from the CD or photocopy this page for your clinical use.

On the probe, present only the untrained exemplars (UT). When the child fails to meet the 90% correct probe criterion, either teach 2 to 4 new exemplars or give additional training trials on already trained stimuli. If needed, select new exemplars for probes. Alternate probes and treatment until the probe criterion is met.

Scripts for Probe Trials

Clinician	[Presents an untrained stimulus] "Whose hat is yellow?"	No modeling or prompts
Child	"Bryce's hat is yellow."	A correct, generalized response
Clinician	Scores the response as correct.	Offers no reinforcement
Clinician	[Presents another untrained stimulus] "Whose antlers are sharp?"	The second probe trial
Child	Moose antlers."	A wrong probe response
Clinician	Scores the response as incorrect.	Offers no corrective feedback

Name:	Date:	Session #:
Age:	**Clinician:**	
Disorder: Language	**Target: Possessive *ez* in sentences (probe)**	
Untrained Stimuli	**Score: + correct; – incorrect or no responses**	
1. Bryce's hat is yellow.		
2. The moose's antlers are sharp.		
3. Denise's pen is purple.		
4. Janice's mittens are warm.		
5. Louise's dog is jumping.		
6. The stewardess's dress is nice.		
7. The goose's feathers are white.		
Percent correct probe (Criterion: 90%)		

When the child meets the 90% correct criterion for the possessive ez in sentences, shift training to other morphologic features or to conversational speech in which the possessive ez is monitored and reinforced.

Irregular Third Person *has*
Irregular Third Person *has* in Phrases
(with Pronoun *she*)

Baserate Protocols

Scripts for Evoked Baserate Trial		Note
Clinician	[showing the picture of a girl holding a black cat] "She has a black cat. Who has a black cat? Start with, *she . . .*"	Prompting the correct initial pronoun
Child	"She."	Scored as a wrong response
Clinician	Scores the response as incorrect.	No corrective feedback
Clinician	[showing the picture of a girl holding two dolls] "She has two dolls. Who has two dolls? Start with, *she . . .*"	The next trial
Child	"She has." ["She has two dolls."]	A correct response
Clinician	Records the response as correct.	No verbal praise

Administer the modeled baserate trials only after completing the evoked trials on all 20 (or more) exemplars.

Scripts for Modeled Baserate Trial		Note
Clinician	[showing the picture of a girl holding a black cat] "She has a black cat. Who has a black cat? Say, *she has.*"	Modeling the target phrase
Child	"She."	A wrong response
Clinician	Records the response as incorrect.	No corrective feedback
Clinician	[showing the picture of a girl holding two dolls] "She has two dolls. Who has two dolls? Say, *she has.*"	Modeling the target phrase
Child	"She has."	A correct response
Clinician	Records the response.	No verbal praise

Baserate at least 20 exemplars as shown on the next page. The phrases may highlight the pronoun + has. However, if the child begins to imitate the whole sentences (e.g., she has a cat), skip the phrase level and move on to the sentence level.

Irregular Third Person *has* in Phrases
(with Pronoun *she*)

Exemplars and Baserate Recording Sheet

Print this page from the CD or photocopy this page for your clinical use.

Name/Age:	Date:
Goal: To establish the baserates of irregular third person *has* (with pronoun *she*) in phrases when asked questions while showing a picture or object.	Clinician:

Clinician's Comments:

Scoring: Correct: ✓   Incorrect or no response: X

Irregular third person *has*	Evoked	Modeled
1. She has [a black cat.]		
2. She has [two dolls.]		
3. She has [a baby brother.]		
4. She has [a big brother.]		
5. She has [a gold fish.]		
6. She has [white bunnies.]		
7. She has [many kites.]		
8. She has [a red book.]		
9. She has [a pink dress.]		
10. She has [a pretty smile.]		
11. She has [many toys.]		
12. She has [a big bed.]		
13. She has [a nice room.]		
14. She has [black shoes.]		
15. She has [many crayons.]		
16. She has [a blue house.]		
17. She has [a shiny ring.]		
18. She has [a big hat.]		
19. She has [a blue jacket.]		
20. She has [a yellow ribbon.]		

After establishing the baserates for the target phrases, initiate treatment. Use the protocols given on the next page

Irregular Third Person *has* in Phrases
(with Pronoun *she*)

Treatment Protocols

Skip this level of training if the child imitates sentences on the modeled baserate trials.

Scripts for Modeled Discrete Trial Training: Irregular third person *has*		Note
Clinician	[showing the picture of a girl holding a black cat] "She has a black cat. Who has a black cat? Say, *she **has**.*"	Vocal emphasis on the target words
Child	"She." ["Has."]	Scored as a wrong response
Clinician	"No, you forgot to say *she **has***. Who has a black cat? Say, *she **has**.*"	Corrective feedback; vocal emphasis on the target word
Child	"She has."	Scored as correct
Clinician	"Very good! You said *she has*!"	Verbal praise

Repeat the trials until the child gives 5 consecutively correct, imitated responses on the exemplar. When the child imitates 5 correct responses in sequence for an exemplar, fade the modeling.

Scripts for Fading the Modeling		Note
Clinician	[showing the picture of a girl holding a black cat] "She has a black cat. Who has a black cat? Say, *she . . .*"	Partial modeling only
Child	"She." ["has."]	A wrong response
Clinician	"No, you forgot to say, ***she has***. who has a black cat? Say, *she . . .*"	Corrective feedback and partial modeling
Child	"She has."	A correct response.
Clinician	"Very good! You said, *she has*!"	Verbal praise
Clinician	"Who has a black cat?"	**An Evoked Trial**
Child	"She has." ["She has a black cat."]	Correct answer
Clinician	"Excellent! You said *she has*!"	Verbal praise

Irregular Third Person *has* in Phrases
(with Pronoun *she*)

Exemplars and Treatment Recording Sheet

Print this page from the CD or photocopy this page for your clinical use.

Name/Age:	Date:
Goal: Production of the irregular third person *has* (with pronoun *she*) in phrases with 90% accuracy when asked questions while showing pictures.	Clinician:

Clinician's Comments:

Scoring: Correct: ✓   Incorrect or no response: X

Target skills	Discrete Trials														
	1	2	3	4	5	6	7	8	9	10	11	12	13	14	15
1. She has [a black cat.]															
2. She has [two dolls.]															
3. She has [a baby brother.]															
4. She has [a big brother.]															
5. She has [a gold fish.]															
6. She has [white bunnies.]															
7. She has [many kites.]															
8. She has [a red book.]															
9. She has [a pink dress.]															
10. She has [a pretty smile.]															

When the child has met the learning criterion of 10 consecutively correct, evoked (nonimitated) responses for each of the 10 target phrases, shift training to the sentence level.

Irregular Third Person *has* in Sentences
(with Pronoun *she*)

Baserate Protocols

Scripts for Evoked Baserate Trial		Note
Clinician	[showing the picture of a girl holding a black cat] "She has a black cat. Who has a black cat? Start with, *she . . .*"	Prompting the correct adverb
Child	"She has." ["She."]	Scored as a wrong response
Clinician	Scores the response as incorrect.	No corrective feedback
Clinician	[showing the picture of a girl holding two dolls] "She has two dolls. Who has two dolls?. Start with, *she . . .*"	The next trial
Child	"She has two dolls."	A correct response
Clinician	Records the response as correct.	No verbal praise

Administer the modeled baserate trials only after completing the evoked trials on all 20 (or more) exemplars.

Scripts for Modeled Baserate Trial		Note
Clinician	[showing the picture of a girl holding a black cat] "She has a black cat. Who has a black cat? Say, *she has a black cat.*"	Modeling the target sentence
Child	"She has." ["One cat."]	A wrong response
Clinician	Records the response as incorrect.	No corrective feedback
Clinician	[showing the picture of a girl holding two dolls] "She has two dolls. Who has two dolls? Say, *she has two dolls.*"	Modeling the target sentence
Child	"She has two dolls."	A correct response
Clinician	Records the response.	No verbal praise

Baserate at least 20 exemplars as shown on the next page.

Irregular Third Person *has* in Sentences
(with Pronoun *she*)

Exemplars and Baserate Recording Sheet

Print this page from the CD or photocopy this page for your clinical use.

Name/Age:	Date:
Goal: To establish the baserates of the irregular third person *has* (with pronoun *she*) in sentences when asked questions while showing a picture or object.	Clinician:

Clinician's Comments:

Scoring: Correct: ✓   Incorrect or no response: X

Irregular third person *has* in Sentences	Evoked	Modeled
1. She has a black cat.		
2. She has two dolls.		
3. She has a baby brother.		
4. She has a big brother.		
5. She has a gold fish.		
6. She has white bunnies.		
7. She has many kites.		
8. She has a red book.		
9. She has a pink dress.		
10. She has a pretty smile.		
11. She has many toys.		
12. She has a big bed.		
13. She has a nice room.		
14. She has black shoes.		
15. She has many crayons.		
16. She has a blue house.		
17. She has a shiny ring.		
18. She has a big hat.		
19. She has a blue jacket.		
20. She has a yellow ribbon.		
Percent correct baserate		

Replace or add new exemplars as you see fit for a given child.

After establishing the baserates for the target sentences, initiate treatment. Use the protocols given on the next page.

Irregular Third Person *has* in Sentences
(with Pronoun *she*)

Treatment Protocols

Scripts for Modeled Discrete Trial Training: Irregular third person *has* (with the pronoun *she*) in sentences		Note
Clinician	[showing the picture of a girl holding a black cat] "She has a black cat. Who has a black cat? Say, ***she has*** *a black cat.*"	Vocal emphasis on the target words
Child	"black cat." ["Has a black cat."]	Scored as a wrong response
Clinician	"No, you forgot to say the whole sentence. Who has a black cat? Say, ***she has*** *a black cat.*"	Corrective feedback; vocal emphasis on the target word
Child	"She has a black cat."	Scored as correct
Clinician	"Very good! You said the whole sentence!"	Verbal praise

Repeat the trials until the child gives 5 consecutively correct, imitated responses on the exemplar. When the child imitates 5 correct responses in sequence for an exemplar, fade the modeling.

Scripts for Fading the Modeling		Note
Clinician	[showing the picture of a girl holding a black cat] "She has a black cat. Who has a black cat? Say, *she . . .*"	Partial modeling only
Child	"Has a black cat." ["She has."]	A wrong response
Clinician	"No, you forgot to say the whole sentence. Who has a black cat? Say, *she . . .*"	Corrective feedback and partial modeling
Child	"She has a black cat."	A correct response
Clinician	"Very good! You said the whole sentence!"	Verbal praise
Clinician	"Who has a black cat?"	**An Evoked Trial**
Child	"She has a black cat."	Correct answer
Clinician	"Excellent! You said, *she has a black cat!*"	Verbal praise

Irregular Third Person *has* in Sentences
(with Pronoun *she*)

Exemplars and Treatment Recording Sheet

Print this page from the CD or photocopy this page for your clinical use.

Name/Age:	Date:
Goal: Production of the irregular third person *has* (with pronoun *she*) in sentences with 90% accuracy when asked questions while showing pictures.	Clinician:

Clinician's Comments:

Scoring: Correct: ✓   Incorrect or no response: X

Target skills	Discrete Trials														
	1	2	3	4	5	6	7	8	9	10	11	12	13	14	15
1. She has a black cat.															
2. She has two dolls.															
3. She has a baby brother.															
4. She has a big brother.															
5. She has a gold fish.															
6. She has white bunnies.															
7. She has many kites.															
8. She has a red book.															
9. She has a pink dress.															
10. She has a pretty smile.															

When the child has met the learning criterion of 10 consecutively correct, evoked (nonimitated) responses for each of the 10 target sentences, conduct a probe. Use the protocols given on the next page.

Irregular Third Person *has* in Sentences
(with Pronoun *she*)

Probe Protocols and Recording Sheet

Print this page from the CD or photocopy this page for your clinical use.

When the child fails to meet the 90% correct probe criterion, teach new exemplars. Probe at least 10 untrained exemplars. Alternate training and probe trials until the child meets the probe criterion.

Scripts for Probe Trials

Clinician	[Presenting an untrained stimulus] "She has many toys. Who has many toys? Start with, *she . . .*"	Prompting the correct response
Child	"She has many toys."	A correct, generalized response
Clinician	Scores the response as correct.	Offers no reinforcement
Clinician	[presents another untrained stimulus] "She has a big bed. Who has a big bed? Start with, *she . . .*"	The second probe trial
Child	"She." ["She has."]	A wrong probe response
Clinician	Scores the response as incorrect.	Offers no corrective feedback

Name:	Date:	Session #:
Age:	Clinician:	
Disorder: Language	Target: Irregular Third Person *has* in Sentences (Probe)	
Untrained Stimuli	Score: + correct; − incorrect or no responses	
1. She has many toys. (UT)		
2. She has a big bed. (UT)		
3. She has a nice room. (UT)		
4. She has black shoes. (UT)		
5. She has many crayons. (UT)		
6. She has a blue house. (UT)		
7. She has a shiny ring. (UT)		
8. She has a big hat. (UT)		
9. She has a blue jacket. (UT)		
10. She has a yellow ribbon. (UT)		
Percent correct probe (Criterion: 90%)		

When the child meets 90% correct probe criterion, teach another target or shift training on the irregular third person has *(with the pronoun* she) *in conversation.*

Irregular Third Person *has* in Phrases
(with Pronoun *he*)

Baserate Protocols

Name/Age:	Date:
Goal: To establish the baserates of the irregular third person *has* (with pronoun *he*) in phrases when asked questions while showing a picture or object.	Clinician:

Scripts for Evoked Baserate Trial		**Note**
Clinician	[showing the picture of a boy playing with a red car] "He has a red car. Who has a red car? Start with, *he . . .* "	Prompting the correct initial pronoun
Child	"He."	Scored as a wrong response
Clinician	Scores the response as incorrect.	No corrective feedback
Clinician	[showing the picture of a boy holding two bats] "He has two bats. Who has two bats? Start with, *he . . .* "	The next trial
Child	"He has." ["He has two bats."]	A correct response
Clinician	Records the response as correct.	No verbal praise

Administer the modeled baserate trials only after completing the evoked trials on all 20 (or more) exemplars.

Scripts for Modeled Baserate Trial		**Note**
Clinician	[showing the picture of a boy playing with a red car] "He has a red car. Who has a red car? Say, *he has.*"	Modeling the target phrase
Child	"He."	A wrong response
Clinician	Records the response as incorrect.	No corrective feedback
Clinician	[showing the picture of a boy holding two bats] "He has two bats. Who has two bats? Say, *he has.*"	Modeling the target phrase
Child	"He has."	A correct response
Clinician	Records the response.	No verbal praise

Baserate at least 20 exemplars as shown on the next page. The phrases may highlight the pronoun + has. However, if the child begins to imitate the whole sentences (e.g., he has a car), skip the phrase level and move on to the sentence level.

Irregular Third Person *has* in Phrases
(with Pronoun *he*)
Exemplars and Baserate Recording Sheet

Print this page from the CD or photocopy this page for your clinical use.

Name/Age:	Date:
Goal: To establish the baserates of the irregular third person *has* (with pronoun *he*) in phrases when asked questions while showing a picture or object.	Clinician:

Clinician's Comments:

Scoring: Correct: ✓   Incorrect or no response: X

Irregular third person *has* with pronoun *he*	Evoked	Modeled
1. He has [a red car.]		
2. He has [two bats.]		
3. He has [a toy train.]		
4. He has [a big sister.]		
5. He has [a brown dog.]		
6. He has [black puppies.]		
7. He has [two bookshelves.]		
8. He has [a many books.]		
9. He has [a blue shirt.]		
10. He has [short hair.]		
11. He has [a funny face.]		
12. He has [a small chair.]		
13. He has [a big closet.]		
14. He has [brown shoes.]		
15. He has [many pictures.]		
16. He has [a green plant.]		
17. He has [a big pen.]		
18. He has [a yellow jacket.]		
19. He has [a pair of boots.]		
20. He has [three hats.]		

Replace or add new exemplars as you see fit for a given child.

After establishing the baserates for the target phrases, initiate treatment. Use the protocols given on the next page.

Irregular Third Person *has* in Phrases
(with Pronoun *he*)

Treatment Protocols

Skip this level of training if the child imitates sentences on the modeled baserate trials.

Scripts for Modeled Discrete Trial Training: Irregular third person *has*		Note
Clinician	[showing the picture of a boy playing with a red car] "He has a red car. Who has a red car? Say, *he has*."	Vocal emphasis on the target words
Child	"He." ["Has."]	Scored as a wrong response
Clinician	"No, you forgot to say *he has*. Who has a red car? Say, *he has*."	Corrective feedback; vocal emphasis on the target word
Child	"He has."	Scored as correct
Clinician	"Very good! You said *he has*!"	Verbal praise

Repeat the trials until the child gives 5 consecutively correct, imitated responses on the exemplar. When the child imitates 5 correct responses in sequence for an exemplar, fade the modeling.

Scripts for Fading the Modeling		Note
Clinician	[showing the picture of a boy playing with a red car] "He has a red car. Who has a red car? Say, *he . . .* "	Partial modeling only
Child	"He." ["has."]	A wrong response
Clinician	"No, you forgot to say *he has*. Who has a red car? Say, *he . . .* "	Corrective feedback and partial modeling
Child	"He has."	A correct response
Clinician	"Very good! You said, *he has*!"	Verbal praise
Clinician	"Who has a red car?"	**An Evoked Trial**
Child	"He has." ["He has a red car."]	Correct answer
Clinician	"Excellent! You said *he has*!"	Verbal praise

Irregular Third Person *has* in Phrases
(with Pronoun *he*)

Exemplars and Treatment Recording Sheet

Print this page from the CD or photocopy this page for your clinical use.

Name/Age:	Date:
Goal: Production of the irregular third person *has* (with pronoun *he*) in phrases with 90% accuracy when asked questions while showing pictures.	Clinician:

Clinician's Comments:

Scoring: Correct: ✓   Incorrect or no response: X

Target skills	Discrete Trials														
	1	2	3	4	5	6	7	8	9	10	11	12	13	14	15
1. He has [a red car.]															
2. He has [two bats.]															
3. He has [a toy train.]															
4. He has [a big sister.]															
5. He has [a brown dog.]															
6. He has [black puppies.]															
7. He has [two bookshelves.]															
8. He has [many books.]															
9. He has [a blue shirt.]															
10. He has [short hair.]															

When the child has met the learning criterion of 10 consecutively correct, evoked (nonimitated) responses for each of the 10 target phrases, shift training to the sentence level.

Irregular Third Person *has* in Sentences
(with Pronoun *he*)

Baserate Protocols

Scripts for Evoked Baserate Trial		Note
Clinician	[showing the picture of a boy playing with a red car] "He has a red car. Who has a red car? Start with, *he* . . ."	Prompting the correct adverb
Child	"He has." ["He."]	Scored as a wrong response
Clinician	Scores the response as incorrect.	No corrective feedback
Clinician	[showing the picture of a boy holding two bats] "He has two bats. Who has two bats?. Start with, *he* . . ."	The next trial
Child	"He has two bats."	A correct response
Clinician	Records the response as correct.	No verbal praise

Administer the modeled baserate trials only after completing the evoked trials on all 20 (or more) exemplars.

Scripts for Modeled Baserate Trial		Note
Clinician	[showing the picture of a boy playing with a red car] "He has a red car. Who has a red car? Say, *he has a red car.*"	Modeling the target sentence
Child	"He has." ["red car."]	A wrong response
Clinician	Records the response as incorrect.	No corrective feedback
Clinician	[showing the picture of a boy holding two bats] "He has two bats. Who has two bats? Say, *he has two bats* . . ."	Modeling the target sentence
Child	"He has two bats."	A correct response
Clinician	Records the response.	No verbal praise

Baserate at least 20 exemplars as shown on the next page.

Irregular Third Person *has* in Sentences (with Pronoun *he*)

Exemplars and Baserate Recording Sheet

Print this page from the CD or photocopy this page for your clinical use.

Name/Age:	Date:
Goal: To establish the baserates of irregular third person *has* (with pronoun *he*) in sentences when asked questions while showing a picture or object.	Clinician:

Clinician's Comments:

Scoring: Correct: ✓ Incorrect or no response: X

Irregular third person *has* in sentences with pronoun *he*	Evoked	Modeled
1. He has a red car.		
2. He has two bats.		
3. He has a toy train.		
4. He has a big sister.		
5. He has a brown dog.		
6. He has black puppies.		
7. He has two bookshelves.		
8. He has a many books.		
9. He has a blue shirt.		
10. He has short hair.		
11. He has a funny face.		
12. He has a small chair.		
13. He has a big closet.		
14. He has brown shoes.		
15. He has many pictures.		
16. He has a green plant.		
17. He has a big pen.		
18. He has a yellow jacket.		
19. He has a pair of boots.		
20. He has three hats.		
Percent correct baserate		

Replace or add new exemplars as you see fit for a given child.

After establishing the baserates for the target sentences, initiate treatment. Use the protocols given on the next page.

Irregular Third Person *has* in Sentences
(with Pronoun *he*)

Treatment Protocols

Scripts for Modeled Discrete Trial Training: Irregular third person *has* in sentences (with the pronoun *he*)		Note
Clinician	[showing the picture of a boy playing a red car] "He has a red car. Who has a red car? Say, ***he has*** *a red car.*"	Vocal emphasis on the target words
Child	"red car." ["Has a red car."]	Scored as a wrong response
Clinician	"No, you forgot to say the whole sentence. Who has a red car? Say, ***he has*** *a red car.*"	Corrective feedback; vocal emphasis on the target word
Child	"He has a red car."	Scored as correct
Clinician	"Very good! You said the whole sentence!"	Verbal praise

Repeat the trials until the child gives 5 consecutively correct, imitated responses on the exemplar. When the child imitates 5 correct responses in sequence for an exemplar, fade the modeling.

Scripts for Fading the Modeling		Note
Clinician	[showing the picture of a boy playing with a red car] "He has a red car. Who has a red car? Say, *he . . .*"	Partial modeling only
Child	"Has a red car." ["He has."]	A wrong response
Clinician	"No, you forgot to say the whole sentence. Who has a red car? Say, *he . . .*"	Corrective feedback and partial modeling
Child	"He has a red car."	A correct response
Clinician	"Very good! You said the whole sentence!"	Verbal praise
Clinician	"Who has a red car?"	**An Evoked Trial**
Child	"He has a red car."	Correct answer
Clinician	"Excellent! You said, *he has a red car!*"	Verbal praise

Irregular Third Person *has* in Sentences
(with Pronoun *he*)

Exemplars and Treatment Recording Sheet

Print this page from the CD or photocopy this page for your clinical use.

Name/Age:	Date:
Goal: Production of the irregular third person *has* (with pronoun *he*) in sentences with 90% accuracy when asked questions while showing pictures.	Clinician:

Clinician's Comments:

Scoring: Correct: ✓   Incorrect or no response: X

Target skills	Discrete Trials														
	1	2	3	4	5	6	7	8	9	10	11	12	13	14	15
1. He has a red car.															
2. He has two bats.															
3. He has a toy train.															
4. He has a big sister.															
5. He has a brown dog.															
6. He has black puppies.															
7. He has two bookshelves.															
8. He has a many books.															
9. He has a blue shirt.															
10. He has short hair.															

When the child has met the learning criterion of 10 consecutively correct, evoked (nonimitated) responses for each of the 10 target sentences, conduct a probe. Use the protocols given on the next page.

Irregular Third Person *has* in Sentences
(with Pronoun *he*)

Probe Protocols and Recording Sheet

Print this page from the CD or photocopy this page for your clinical use.

When the child fails to meet the 90% correct probe criterion, teach new exemplars. Probe at least 10 untrained exemplars. Alternate training and probe trials until the child meets the probe criterion.

Scripts for Probe Trials

Clinician	[Presenting an untrained stimulus] "He has a funny face. Who has a funny face? Start with, *he* . . ."	Prompting the correct response
Child	"He has a funny face."	A correct, generalized response
Clinician	Scores the response as correct.	Offers no reinforcement
Clinician	[presents another untrained stimulus] "He has a small chair. Who has small chair? Start with, *he* . . ."	The second probe trial
Child	"He." ["He has."]	A wrong probe response
Clinician	Scores the response as incorrect.	Offers no corrective feedback

Name:		Date:	Session #:
Age:		Clinician:	
Disorder: Language		Target: Irregular Third Person *has* in Sentences (Probe)	
Untrained Stimuli		**Score: + correct; – incorrect or no responses**	
1. He has a funny face. (UT)			
2. He has a small chair. (UT)			
3. He has a big closet. (UT)			
4. He has brown shoes. (UT)			
5. He has many pictures. (UT)			
6. He has a green plant. (UT)			
7. He has a big pen. (UT)			
8. He has a yellow jacket. (UT)			
9. He has a pair of boots. (UT)			
10. He has three hats. (UT)			
Percent correct probe (Criterion: 90%)			

When the child meets 90% correct probe criterion, teach another target or shift training on the irregular third person has *with the pronoun* he *in conversation.*

Irregular Third Person *have* in Sentences
(with Pronoun *they*)

Baserate Protocols

Scripts for Evoked Baserate Trial		Note
Clinician	[showing the picture of several people and multiple cats] "They have cats. What do they have? Start with, *they* . . ."	Prompting the correct adverb
Child	"Cats." ["They."]	Scored as a wrong response
Clinician	Scores the response as incorrect.	No corrective feedback
Clinician	[showing the picture of several people and multiple cars] "They have cars. What do they have? Start with, *they* . . ."	The next trial
Child	"They have cars."	A correct response
Clinician	Records the response as correct.	No verbal praise

Administer the modeled baserate trials only after completing the evoked trials on all 20 (or more) exemplars.

Scripts for Modeled Baserate Trial		Note
Clinician	[showing the picture of several people and multiple cats] "They have cats. What do they have? Say, *they have cats.*"	Modeling the target sentence
Child	"Cats." ["They have"]	A wrong response
Clinician	Records the response as incorrect.	No corrective feedback
Clinician	[showing the picture of several people and multiple cars] "They have cars. What do they have? Say, *they have cars.*"	Modeling the target sentence
Child	"They have cars."	A correct response
Clinician	Records the response.	No verbal praise

Baserate at least 20 exemplars as shown on the next page.

Irregular Third Person *have* in Sentences
(with Pronoun *they*)

Exemplars and Baserate Recording Sheet

Print this page from the CD or photocopy this page for your clinical use.

Name/Age:	Date:
Goal: To establish the baserates of the irregular third person *have* (with pronoun *they*) in sentences when asked questions while showing a picture or object.	Clinician:

Clinician's Comments:

Scoring: Correct: ✓   Incorrect or no response: X

Irregular third person *has* in sentences with pronoun *they*	Evoked	Modeled
1. They have cats.		
2. They have cars.		
3. They have houses.		
4. They have children.		
5. They have dogs.		
6. They have trees.		
7. They have flowers.		
8. They have televisions.		
9. They have books.		
10. They have toys.		
11. They have gold fish.		
12. They have a blackboard.		
13. They have a teacher.		
14. They have jackets.		
15. They have desks.		
16. They have chairs.		
17. They have computers.		
18. They have pencils.		
19. They have a map.		
20. They have a globe.		
Percent correct bascrate		

Replace or add new exemplars as you see fit for a given child.

After establishing the baserates for the target sentences, initiate treatment. Use the protocols given on the next page.

Irregular Third Person *have* in Sentences
(with Pronoun *they*)

Treatment Protocols

Scripts for Modeled Discrete Trial Training: Irregular third person *have* in sentences with pronoun *they*		Note
Clinician	[showing the picture of several people and multiple cats] "They have cats. What do they have? Say, **they have** cats."	Vocal emphasis on the target words
Child	"Cats." ["Have cats."]	Scored as a wrong response
Clinician	"No, you forgot to say the whole sentence. What do they have? Say, **they have** cats."	Corrective feedback; vocal emphasis on the target word
Child	"They have cats."	Scored as correct
Clinician	"Very good! You said the whole sentence!"	Verbal praise

Repeat the trials until the child gives 5 consecutively correct, imitated responses on the exemplar. When the child imitates 5 correct responses in sequence for an exemplar, fade the modeling.

Scripts for Fading the Modeling		Note
Clinician	[showing the picture of several people and multiple cats] "They have cats. What do they have? Say, *they* . . ."	Partial modeling only
Child	"They." ["Have cats."]	A wrong response
Clinician	"No, you forgot to say the whole sentence. What do they have? Say, *they* . . ."	Corrective feedback and partial modeling
Child	"They have cats."	A correct response.
Clinician	"Very good! You said the whole sentence!"	Verbal praise
Clinician	"What do they have?"	**An Evoked Trial**
Child	"They have cats."	Correct answer
Clinician	"Excellent! You said, *they have cats!*"	Verbal praise

Irregular Third Person *have* in Sentences
(with Pronoun *they*)

Exemplars and Treatment Recording Sheet

Print this page from the CD or photocopy this page for your clinical use.

Name/Age:	Date:
Goal: Production of the irregular third person *have* (with pronoun *they*) in sentences with 90% accuracy when asked questions while showing pictures.	Clinician:

Clinician's Comments:

Scoring: Correct: ✓   Incorrect or no response: X

Target skills	Discrete Trials														
	1	2	3	4	5	6	7	8	9	10	11	12	13	14	15
1. They have cats.															
2. They have cars.															
3. They have houses.															
4. They have children.															
5. They have dogs.															
6. They have trees.															
7. They have flowers.															
8. They have televisions.															
9. They have books.															
10. They have toys.															

When the child has met the learning criterion of 10 consecutively correct, evoked (nonimitated) responses for each of the 10 target sentences, conduct a probe. Use the protocols given on the next page.

Irregular Third Person *have* in Sentences
(with Pronoun *they*)

Probe Protocols and Recording Sheet

Print this page from the CD or photocopy this page for your clinical use.

When the child fails to meet the 90% correct probe criterion, teach new exemplars. Probe at least 10 untrained exemplars. Alternate training and probe trials until the child meets the probe criterion.

Scripts for Probe Trials

Clinician	[Presenting an untrained stimulus] "They have gold fish. What do they have? Start with, *they* . . ."	Prompting the correct response
Child	"They have goldfish."	A correct, generalized response
Clinician	Scores the response as correct.	Offers no reinforcement
Clinician	[presents another untrained stimulus] "They have a blackboard. What do they have? Start with, *they* . . ."	The second probe trial
Child	"They." ["blackboard."]	A wrong probe response
Clinician	Scores the response as incorrect.	Offers no corrective feedback

Name:	Date:	Session #:
Age:	**Clinician:**	
Disorder: Language	**Target: Irregular Third Person *have* in Sentences (Probe)**	
Untrained Stimuli	**Score: + correct; – incorrect or no responses**	
1. They have goldfish. (UT)		
2. They have a blackboard. (UT)		
3. They have a teacher. (UT)		
4. They have jackets. (UT)		
5. They have desks. (UT)		
6. They have chairs. (UT)		
7. They have computers. (UT)		
8. They have pencils. (UT)		
9. They have a map. (UT)		
10. They have a globe. (UT)		
Percent correct probe (Criterion: 90%)		

When the child meets 90% correct probe criterion, teach another target or shift training on the irregular third person have *with the pronoun* they *in conversation.*

Prepositions

Overview

Prepositions *in* and *on* are grammatic morphemes that children master relatively early. In Brown's (1973) longitudinal study of three children, these two prepositions were the second and third morphemes to reach the mastery criterion. Prepositions are important in expressing spatial relations and are essential in expanding verbal skills. Children with language disorders need training in the correct use of prepositions.

Prepositions *in* and *on* are relatively easy to master (Brown, 1973; Gleason, 2001; McLaughlin, 1998), and perhaps equally easy to teach children with language disorders. Other prepositions (e.g., *behind, beside, in front of*) are relatively more difficult to master. Nonetheless, all prepositions allow concrete representations during teaching, and hence are eminently teachable.

General Training Strategy

Although pictures may be fine in teaching prepositions, objects that can be manipulated to show the spatial relationships may be the most effective. Objects placed *on, in, under*, and *behind* other objects are more easy to see. Such concrete operations may promote more active learning, especially when the child is asked to manipulate objects and their spatial relationships during treatment. The first 6 to 8 exemplars taught may use object manipulations. Probe may involve pictures that show spatial relations that are not practical to manipulate in clinical sessions (e.g., *fish in the water, boy in the bed*).

The phrase level baserating and teaching protocols are provided and may be needed in many cases. However, for some children who imitate the prepositions in sentences, this initial level of training may be skipped. In such cases, the training may be started with simple sentences that include various prepositions.

Preposition *in*
Preposition *in* in Phrases

Baserate Protocols

At the beginning of each trial, help the child perform the required action. For instance, have the child place a doll inside a toy house. Keep the objects in full sight of the child as you administer the baserate and treatment trials. Before asking the relevant questions ("where is the [noun]" in most cases), point to the object that is inside something.

Administer the evoked trials first followed by modeled trials. Do not provide feedback on any trials; just record the child's responses on the recording sheet provided on the next page or printed from the CD.

Note: *The target phrases include the definite article. The clinician models the phrase with the article, but does not emphasize it or provide contingent consequences (reinforcement or corrective feedback) for it. A child may or may not produce the article. Score the responses solely on the basis of presence or absence of the preposition. Do not score it incorrect if the child fails to produce the article as it is not the target in this segment of teaching.*

Scripts for Evoked Baserate Trial		Note
Clinician	[after the child has placed a doll inside a toy house] "Where is the doll?"	No modeling
Child	"House." ["box"]	A wrong response
Clinician	Records the response as incorrect.	No corrective feedback
Clinician	[after the child has placed a key in a small bucket] "Where is the key?"	The next trial
Child	"In bucket." ["In the bucket"]	A correct response; the omission of the article and the noun is ignored
Clinician	Records the response as correct.	No verbal praise

Administer the modeled baserate trials only after completing the evoked trials on all 20 (or more) exemplars. Again, let the child perform the required actions before starting each trial.

Scripts for Modeled Baserate Trial		Note
Clinician	"The doll is in the house. Where is the doll? Say, *doll in the house.*"	Modeling
Child	"House."	A wrong response
Clinician	Records the response as incorrect.	No corrective feedback
Clinician	"The key is in the bucket. Where is the key? Say, *key in the bucket.*"	Modeling
Child	"Key in bucket." ["In the bucket"]	A correct response; omission of the article is ignored
Clinician	Records the response.	No verbal praise

Baserate at least 20 exemplars as shown on the next page.

Preposition *in* in Phrases

Exemplars and Baserate Recording Sheet

Print this page from the CD or photocopy this page for your clinical use.

Name/Age:	Date:
Goal: To establish the baserates of phrases with the preposition *in* when asked questions while showing a picture or object.	Clinician:

Clinician's Comments:

Scoring: Correct: ✓   Incorrect or no response: X

Phrases with Preposition *in*	Evoked	Modeled
1. Doll in the house		
2. Key in the bucket		
3. Pencil in the mug		
4. Car in the box		
5. Book in the basket		
6. Toy in the store		
7. Phone in the bag		
8. Chair in the room		
9. Fish in the water		
10. Water in the cup		
11. Boy in the bed		
12. Cookie in the jar		
13. Soup in the pot		
14. Pig in the farm		
15. Tiger in the zoo		
16. Slide in the park		
17. Cat in the hat		
18. Dog in the car		
19. Kitty in the shoe		
20. Table in the room		
Percent correct baserate		

Replace or add exemplars as you see fit for the child.

After establishing the baserates of preposition in *(in phrases), begin teaching them. Use the protocols given on the next page.*

Preposition *in* in Phrases

Treatment Protocols

At the beginning of each trial, have the child place a target object inside a container. (e.g., have the child place a small doll inside a toy house). Each time, point to the target object inside the container.

Scripts for Modeled Discrete Trial Training		Note
Clinician	"The doll is in the house. Where is the doll? Say, *doll **in** the house.*"	Vocal emphasis on the target morpheme
Client	"House."	A wrong response
Clinician	"No, that is not correct. Where is the doll? Say, *doll **in** the house.*"	Corrective feedback; vocal emphasis on the preposition
Client	"doll in house." ["In the house."]	A correct response
Clinician	"Very good! You said doll **in** house!"	Verbal praise

Repeat the trials until the child gives 5 consecutively correct, imitated responses. When the child imitates 5 correct responses in sequence, fade the modeling. Always point to the target object before asking a question.

Scripts for Fading the Modeling		Note
Clinician	"The doll is in the house. Where is the doll? Say, *doll is . . .*"	Partial modeling only
Client	"House."	A wrong response
Clinician	"No, that is not correct. Doll is in the house. Where is the doll? Say, *the doll . . .*"	Corrective feedback and partial modeling
Client	"doll in house." ["Doll in the house."]	A correct response
Clinician	"Very good! You said *doll in house!*"	Verbal praise
Clinician	"Where is the doll?"	**An Evoked Trial**
Client	"Doll in house." ["Doll in the house."]	Correct answer

If the wrong responses persist on 4 to 5 evoked trials, reinstate partial or full modeling for a few trials, again fade the modeling, and re-present the evoked trials.

When the child meets the tentative learning criterion of 10 consecutively correct, nonimitated responses for a given exemplar, move on to the next exemplar. With this procedure, teach 6 to 8 exemplars. Use different exemplars as you see fit for a given child. Use the exemplars and the recording sheet given on the next page (or copy it from the CD).

Preposition *in* in Phrases

Exemplars and Treatment Recording Sheet

Print this page from the CD or photocopy this page for your clinical use.

Name/Age:	Date:
Goal: Production of phrases with the proposition *in* with 90% accuracy when asked questions while showing pictures.	Clinician:

Clinician's Comments:

Scoring: Correct: ✓ Incorrect or no response: X

Target skills	Discrete Trials														
	1	2	3	4	5	6	7	8	9	10	11	12	13	14	15
1. Doll in the house															
2. Key in the bucket															
3. Pencil in the mug															
4. Car in the box															
5. Book in the basket															
6. Toy in the store															
7. Phone in the bag															
8. Chair in the room															

Teach 6 to 8 exemplars each to a training criterion of 10 consecutively correct, nonimitated responses. When the child meets this criterion, begin teaching sentences with the target preposition. Before starting treatment, baserate the production of the preposition in sentences.

Preposition *in* in Sentences

Baserate Protocols

At the beginning of each trial, ask the child to place an object inside a container. Point to the object inside and then ask the specified question. Do not respond in any way to the child's correct, incorrect, or lack of responses.

Scripts for Evoked Baserate Trial		Note
Clinician	[after the child has placed a doll inside a toy house] "Where is the doll? Start with, *doll is . . .*"	Prompting the sentence form
Child	"House."	A wrong response
Clinician	Records the response as incorrect.	No corrective feedback
Clinician	[after the child has placed a key in a small bucket] "Where is the key? Start with, *key is . . .*"	The next trial
Child	"In bucket." ["In the bucket"]	Scored as incorrect because the child did not produce the sentence.
Clinician	Records the response as incorrect.	No verbal praise

Administer the modeled baserate trials only after completing the evoked trials on all 20 (or more) exemplars. Again, let the child perform the required actions before starting each trial.

Scripts for Modeled Baserate Trial		Note
Clinician	"The doll is in the house. Where is the doll? Say, *doll is in the house.*"	Modeling
Child	"In house."	Scored as a wrong response
Clinician	Records the response as incorrect.	No corrective feedback
Clinician	"The key is in the bucket. Where is the key? Say, *key is in the bucket.*"	Modeling
Child	"Key is in bucket." ["Key is in bucket"]	A correct response; omission of the article is ignored
Clinician	Records the response.	No verbal praise

Baserate at least 20 exemplars as shown on the next page.

Preposition *in* in Sentences

Exemplars and Baserate Recording Sheet

Print this page from the CD or photocopy this page for your clinical use.

Name/Age:	Date:
Goal: To establish the baserates of sentences with the preposition *in* when asked questions while showing a picture or object.	Clinician:

Clinician's Comments:

Scoring: Correct: ✓ Incorrect or no response: X

Sentence Level	Evoked	Modeled
1. Doll is in the house.		
2. Key is in the bucket.		
3. Pencil is in the mug.		
4. Car is in the box.		
5. Book is in the basket.		
6. Toy is in the store.		
7. Phone is in the bag.		
8. Chair is in the room.		
9. Fish is in the water.		
10. Water is in the cup.		
11. Boy is in the bed.		
12. Cookie is in the jar.		
13. Soup is in the pot.		
14. Pig is in the farm.		
15. Tiger is in the zoo.		
16. Slide is in the park.		
17. Cat is in the hat.		
18. Dog is in the car.		
19. Kitty is in the shoe.		
20. Table is in the room.		
Percent correct baserate		

Replace or add new exemplars as you see fit for a given child.

After establishing the baserates for the target preposition in *in sentences, initiate treatment. Use the protocols given on the next page.*

Preposition *in* in Sentences

Treatment Protocols

Teach 6 to 8 sentences with the preposition in *in sentences using the following script.*

Have the child perform the required action before starting treatment. Each time, point to the target objects.

Scripts for Modeled Discrete Trial Training		Note
Clinician	"The doll is in the house. Where is the doll? Say, **the doll is in** the house."	Vocal emphasis on the target words; article *the* is added, but considered optional.
Client	"In house." ["In the house."]	Scored as a wrong response
Clinician	"No, You didn't say the whole sentence. Where is the doll? Say, **the doll is in** the house."	Corrective feedback; vocal emphasis on the target words
Client	"The doll is in house." ["Doll is in the house."]	Scored as correct; one or more article may be included
Clinician	"Very good! You said **the doll is in** house!"	Verbal praise

Repeat the trials until the child gives 5 consecutively correct, imitated responses. When the child imitates 5 correct responses in sequence, fade the modeling. Always point to the target object before asking a question.

Scripts for Fading the Modeling		Note
Clinician	"The doll is in the house. Where is the doll? Say, the *doll is . . .* "	Partial modeling only
Client	"House."	A wrong response
Clinician	"No, you didn't say the whole sentence. *The doll is in the house.* Where is the doll? Say, *the doll is . . .* "	Corrective feedback and partial modeling
Client	"The doll is in house." ["Doll is in the house."]	A correct response; optional article production
Clinician	"Very good! You said, *the doll is in house!*"	Verbal praise
Clinician	"Where is the doll?"	**An Evoked Trial**
Client	"The doll is in house." ["Doll is in the house; The doll is in the house."]	Correct answer
Clinician	"Excellent! You said the whole sentence!"	Verbal praise

Preposition *in* in Sentences

Exemplars and Treatment Recording Sheet

Print this page from the CD or photocopy this page for your clinical use.

Name/Age:	Date:
Goal: Production of the proposition *in* in sentences with 90% accuracy when asked questions while showing pictures.	Clinician:

Clinician's Comments:

Scoring: Correct: ✓   Incorrect or no response: X

Target skills	Discrete Trials														
	1	2	3	4	5	6	7	8	9	10	11	12	13	14	15
1. Doll is in the house															
2. Key is in the bucket															
3. Pencil is in the mug															
4. Car is in the box															
5. Book is in the basket															
6. Toy is in the store															
7. Phone is in the bag															
8. Chair is in the room															

When the child has met the learning criterion 10 consecutively correct, evoked (nonimitated) responses for each of the 6 to 8 target sentences, conduct a probe to see if the production of the preposition has generalized to previously baserated but untrained sentences. Use the protocol given on the next page (or print it from the CD).

Preposition *in* in Sentences

Probe Protocols and Recording Sheet

Print this page from the CD or photocopy this page for your clinical use.

On the probes, present only the untrained exemplars (UT). When the child fails to meet the 90% correct probe criterion, either teach 2 to 4 new exemplars or give additional training trials on already trained exemplars. If needed, select new exemplars for probes. Probe at least 10 untrained exemplars. Alternate probes and treatment until the probe criterion is met.

Scripts for Probe Trials

Clinician	[Presents an untrained stimulus] "Where is the fish?"	No modeling or prompts
Child	"The fish is in the water."	A correct, generalized response
Clinician	Scores the response as correct.	Offers no reinforcement
Clinician	[Presents another untrained stimulus] "Where is the water?"	The second probe trial
Child	"Cup." ["In cup."]	A wrong probe response
Clinician	Scores the response as incorrect.	Offers no corrective feedback

Name:	Date:	Session #:
Age:	**Clinician:**	
Disorder: Language	**Target Behavior: Preposition *in* in sentences (probe)**	

Untrained Stimuli	Score: + correct; – incorrect or no responses
1. Fish is in the water. (UT)	
2. Water is in the cup. (UT)	
3. Boy is in the bed. (UT)	
4. Cookie is in the jar. (UT)	
5. Soup is in the pot. (UT)	
6. Pig is in the farm. (UT)	
7. Tiger is in the zoo. (UT)	
8. Slide is in the park. (UT)	
9. Cat is in the hat. (UT)	
10. Dog is in the car. (UT)	
11. Kitty is in the shoe. (UT)	
12. Table is in the room. (UT)	
Percent correct probe (Criterion: 90%)	

If the child does not meet the probe criterion, give additional training on already trained sentences and subsequently readminister the probe trials. When the child meets the 90% correct sentence probe criterion for the preposition in, *shift training to other morphologic features (such as the preposition* on *as shown next) or to conversational speech in which the preposition is monitored and reinforced.*

Preposition *on*
Preposition *on* in Phrases
Baserate Protocols

At the beginning of each trial, help the child perform the required action. For instance, have the child place a toy car on the rug. Keep the objects in full sight of the child as you administer the baserate and treatment trials. Before asking the relevant questions ("where is the [noun]" in most cases), point to the object that is on something. Some exemplars need to be taught with pictures. In such cases, point to the picture at the beginning of each trial.

Administer the evoked trials first followed by modeled trials. Do not provide feedback on any trials; just record the responses on the recording sheet provided on the next page or printed from the CD.

Note: *The target phrases include the definite article. The clinician models the phrase with the article, but does not emphasize it or provide contingent consequences (reinforcement or corrective feedback) for it. A child may or may not produce the article. Score the responses solely on the basis of presence or absence of the preposition. Do not score it incorrect if the child fails to produce the article as it is not the target in this segment of teaching.*

Scripts for Evoked Baserate Trial		Note
Clinician	[after the child has placed a car on the rug] "Where is the car?"	No modeling
Child	"Rug." ["Floor"]	A wrong response
Clinician	Records the response as incorrect.	No corrective feedback
Clinician	[after the child has placed a toy dog on the hood of a toy car] "Where is the dog?"	The next trial
Child	"On hood." ["On car"]	A correct response; the omission of the article is ignored
Clinician	Records the response as correct.	No verbal praise

Administer the modeled baserate trials only after completing the evoked trials on all 20 (or more) exemplars. Again, let the child perform the required actions before starting each trial.

Scripts for Modeled Baserate Trial		Note
Clinician	"The car is on the rug. Where is the car? Say, *on the rug.*"	Modeling
Child	"Rug."	A wrong response
Clinician	Records the response as incorrect.	No corrective feedback
Clinician	"The dog is on the hood. Where is the dog? Say, *on the hood.*"	Modeling
Child	"On hood." ["on car"]	A correct response; omission of the article is ignored
Clinician	Records the response.	No verbal praise

Baserate at least 20 exemplars as shown on the next page.

Preposition *on* in Phrases

Exemplars and Baserate Recording Sheet

Print this page from the CD or photocopy this page for your clinical use.

Name/Age:	Date:
Goal: To establish the baserates of the preposition *on* in phrases when asked questions while showing a picture or object.	Clinician:

Clinician's Comments:

Scoring: Correct: ✓   Incorrect or no response: X

Preposition *on* in phrases	Evoked	Modeled
1. on the rug.		
2. on the hood.		
3. on the chair.		
4. on the floor.		
5. on the table.		
6. on the box.		
7. on the floor.		
8. on the shelf.		
9. on the swing.		
10. on the roof.		
11. on the wall.		
12. on the head.		
13. on the hill.		
14. on the paper.		
15. on the tree.		
16. on the slide.		
17. on the bike.		
18. on the plate.		
19. on the grass.		
20. on the table.		
Percent correct baserate		

Replace or add exemplars as you see fit to suit an individual child. Consider the article in the exemplars as optional. After establishing the baserates, initiate treatment. Use the protocols that follow.

Preposition *on* in Phrases

Treatment Protocols

Use various toy objects that the child could place on other objects. Use pictures for exemplars that cannot be represented concretely.

At the beginning of each trial, have the child place a target object on another object. (e.g., have the child place a coat on a chair). Each time, point to the target object.

Scripts for Modeled Discrete Trial Training		Note
Clinician	"The car is on the rug. Where is the car? Say, **on** *the rug.*"	Vocal emphasis on the target morpheme
Client	"Rug."	A wrong response
Clinician	"No, that is not correct. Where is the car? Say, **on** *the rug.*"	Corrective feedback; vocal emphasis on the target word
Client	"On rug." ["On the rug."]	A correct response
Clinician	"Very good! You said **on** *rug*!"	Verbal praise

Repeat the trials until the child gives 5 consecutively correct, imitated responses. When the child imitates 5 correct responses in sequence, fade the modeling. Always point to the target object before asking a question.

Scripts for Fading the Modeling		Note
Clinician	"The car is on the rug. Where is the car? Say, *car is . . .*"	Partial modeling only
Client	"Rug."	A wrong response
Clinician	"No, that is not correct. Car is on the rug. Where is the car? Say, *the car is . . .*"	Corrective feedback and partial modeling
Client	"On rug." ["On the rug."]	A correct response
Clinician	"Very good! You said *on rug*!"	Verbal praise
Clinician	"Where is the car?"	**An Evoked Trial**
Client	"On rug." ["On the rug."]	Correct answer

If the wrong responses persist on 4 to 5 evoked trials, reinstate partial or full modeling for a few trials, again fade the modeling, and re-present the evoked trials.

When the child meets the tentative learning criterion of 10 consecutively correct, nonimitated responses for a given exemplar, move on to the next exemplar. With this procedure, teach 6 to 8 exemplars. Use different exemplars as you see fit for a given child. Use the exemplars given on the next page (or copy it from the CD).

Preposition *on* in Phrases

Exemplars and Treatment Recording Sheet

Print this page from the CD or photocopy this page for your clinical use.

Name/Age:	Date:
Goal: Production of the proposition *on* in phrases with 90% accuracy when asked questions while showing pictures.	Clinician:

Clinician's Comments:

Scoring: Correct: ✓   Incorrect or no response: X

Target skills	Discrete Trials														
	1	2	3	4	5	6	7	8	9	10	11	12	13	14	15
1. on the rug															
2. on the hood															
3. on the chair															
4. on the floor															
5. on the table															
6. on the box															
7. on the floor															
8. on the shelf															

Teach 6 to 8 exemplars each to a training criterion of 10 consecutively correct, nonimitated responses. Then, shift training to the sentence level. Before teaching the preposition in sentences, baserate their production.

Preposition *on* in Sentences

Baserate Protocols

At the beginning of each trial, either ask the child to place an object on something or show a relevant picture. Point to the object and then ask the specified question. Do not respond in any way to the child's correct, incorrect, or lack of responses.

Scripts for Evoked Baserate Trial		Note
Clinician	"Where is the car?"	No modeling
Child	"Rug." ["box"]	A wrong response
Clinician	Records the response as incorrect.	No corrective feedback
Clinician	"Where is the dog?"	The next trial
Child	"On hood." ["On the hood"]	Scored as incorrect because the child did not produce the sentence
Clinician	Records the response as incorrect.	No corrective feedback

Administer the modeled baserate trials only after completing the evoked trials on all 20 (or more) exemplars. Again, let the child perform the required actions before starting each trial.

Scripts for Modeled Baserate Trial		Note
Clinician	"The car is on the rug. Where is the car? Say, *the car is on the rug.*"	Modeling
Child	"On rug." ["On the rug."]	Scored as a wrong response
Clinician	Records the response as incorrect.	No corrective feedback
Clinician	"The dog is on the hood. Where is the dog? Say, *the dog is on the hood.*"	Modeling
Child	"Dog is on hood."	A correct response; omission of the article is ignored
Clinician	Records the response.	No verbal praise

Baserate at least 20 exemplars as shown on the next page.

Preposition *on* in Sentences
Exemplars and Baserate Recording Sheet

Print this page from the CD or photocopy this page for your clinical use.

Name/Age:		Date:
Goal: To establish the baserates of preposition *on* in sentences when asked questions while showing a picture or object.		Clinician:

Clinician's Comments:

Scoring: Correct: ✓   Incorrect or no response: X

Preposition *on* in Sentences	Evoked	Modeled
1. The car is on the rug.		
2. The dog is on the hood.		
3. The coat is on the chair.		
4. The bug is on the floor.		
5. The ball is on the table.		
6. The cat is on the box.		
7. The bag is on the floor.		
8. The book is on the shelf.		
9. The boy is on the swing.		
10. The bird is on the roof.		
11. The clock is on the wall.		
12. The hat is on the head.		
13. The tree is on the hill.		
14. The sticker is on the paper.		
15. The monkey is on the tree.		
16. The girl is on the slide.		
17. The man is on the bike.		
18. The food is on the plate.		
19. The frog is on the grass.		
20. The flower is on the table.		
Percent correct baserate		

Replace or add new exemplars as you see fit for a given child.

After establishing the baserates for the target preposition in sentences, initiate treatment. Use the protocols given on the next page.

Preposition *on* in Sentences
Treatment Protocols

Teach 6 to 8 sentences with the preposition on *in sentences using the following script.*

Have the child perform the required action before starting treatment or show a relevant picture. Each time, point to the target objects.

Scripts for Modeled Discrete Trial Training		Note
Clinician	"The car is on the rug. Where is the car? Say, ***the car is on** the rug*."	Vocal emphasis on the target words
Client	"On house." ["On the house."]	Scored as a wrong response
Clinician	"No, You didn't say the whole sentence. Where is the car? Say, ***the car is on** the rug*."	Corrective feedback; vocal emphasis on the target words
Client	"Car is on rug." ["Car is on the rug."]	Scored as correct; one or more article may be included
Clinician	"Very good! You said ***the car is on** rug*!"	Verbal praise

Repeat the trials until the child gives 5 consecutively correct, imitated responses. When the child imitates 5 correct responses in sequence, fade the modeling. Always point to the target object before asking a question.

Scripts for Fading the Modeling		Note
Clinician	"The car is on the rug. Where is the car? Say, *the car is . . .*"	Partial modeling only
Client	"Rug."	A wrong response
Clinician	"No, you didn't say the whole sentence. *The car is on the rug.* Where is the car? Say, *the car is . . .*"	Corrective feedback and partial modeling
Client	"The car is on rug." ["Car is on the rug."]	A correct response; optional article production
Clinician	"Very good! You said, *the car is on rug*!"	Verbal praise
Clinician	"Where is the car?"	**An Evoked Trial**
Client	"The car is on rug." ["Car is on the rug; The car is on the rug."]	Correct answer
Clinician	"Excellent! You said the whole sentence!"	Verbal praise

Preposition *on* in Sentences

Exemplars and Treatment Recording Sheet

Print this page from the CD or photocopy this page for your clinical use.

Name/Age:	Date:
Goal: Production of the proposition *on* in sentences with 90% accuracy when asked questions while showing pictures.	Clinician:

Clinician's Comments:

Scoring: Correct: ✓   Incorrect or no response: X

Target skills	Discrete Trials														
	1	2	3	4	5	6	7	8	9	10	11	12	13	14	15
1. The car is on the rug.															
2. The dog is on the hood.															
3. The coat is on the chair.															
4. The bug is on the floor.															
5. The ball is on the table.															
6. The cat is on the box.															
7. The bag is on the floor.															
8. The book is on the shelf.															

When the child has met the learning criterion 10 consecutively correct, evoked (nonimitated) responses for each of the 6 to 8 target sentences, conduct a probe to see if the production of the preposition has generalized to previously baserated but untrained sentences.

Use the protocol given on the next page (or print it from the CD).

Preposition *on* in Sentences

Probe Protocols and Recording Sheet

Print this page from the CD or photocopy this page for your clinical use.

On the probes, present only the untrained exemplars (UT). When the child fails to meet the 90% correct probe criterion, either teach 2 to 4 new exemplars or give additional training trials on already trained exemplars. If needed, select new exemplars for probes. Probe at least 10 untrained exemplars. Alternate probes and treatment until the probe criterion is met.

Scripts for Probe Trials

Clinician	[Presents an untrained stimulus] "Where is the boy?"	No modeling or prompts
Child	"The boy is on the swing."	A correct, generalized response
Clinician	Scores the response as correct.	Offers no reinforcement
Clinician	[Presents another untrained stimulus] "Where is the bird?"	The second probe trial
Child	"Roof." ["on roof."]	A wrong probe response
Clinician	Scores the response as incorrect.	Offers no corrective feedback

Name:	Date:	Session #:
Age:	**Clinician:**	
Disorder: Language	**Target Behavior: Preposition *on* in sentences (probe)**	
Untrained Stimuli	**Score: + correct; – incorrect or no responses**	
1. The boy is on the swing (UT).		
2. The bird is on the roof (UT).		
3. The clock is on the wall (UT).		
4. The hat is on the head(UT).		
5. The tree is on the hill (UT).		
6. The sticker is on the paper (UT).		
7. The monkey is on the tree (UT).		
8. The girl is on the slide (UT).		
9. The man is on the bike (UT).		
10. The food is on the plate (UT).		
11. The frog is on the grass (UT).		
12. The flower is on the table (UT).		
Percent correct probe (Criterion: 90%)		

If the child does not meet the probe criterion, give additional training on already trained sentences and subsequently readminister the probe trials. When the child meets the 90% correct sentence probe criterion for the preposition on, shift training to other morphologic features (such as the preposition under as shown next) or to conversational speech in which the preposition is monitored and reinforced.

Preposition *under*
Preposition *under* in Phrases

Baserate Protocols

When practical, help the child perform the required action. For instance, have the child place a doll under the table. Let the object that lies under something be at least partially visible to the child throughout the teaching session. Point to the object. When this is not possible, use realistic pictures and point to the object or person under something before asking the relevant question.

Administer the evoked trials first followed by modeled trials. Do not provide feedback on any trials; just record the responses on the recording sheet provided on the next page or printed from the CD.

Note: *The target phrases include the definite article. The clinician models the phrase with the article, but does not emphasize it or provide contingent consequences (reinforcement or corrective feedback) for it. A child may or may not produce the article. Score the responses solely on the basis of presence or absence of the preposition. Do not score it incorrect if the child fails to produce the article as it is not the target in this segment of teaching.*

Scripts for Evoked Baserate Trial		Note
Clinician	[after the child has placed a doll under the table] "Where is the doll?"	No modeling
Child	"Table."	A wrong response
Clinician	Records the response as incorrect.	No corrective feedback
Clinician	[after the child has placed a toy car under a hat] "Where is the car?"	The next trial
Child	"Under hat."	A correct response; the omission of the article is ignored
Clinician	Records the response as correct.	No verbal praise

Administer the modeled baserate trials only after completing the evoked trials on all 20 (or more) exemplars. Again, let the child perform the required actions before starting each trial.

Scripts for Modeled Baserate Trial		Note
Clinician	"The doll is under the table. Where is the doll? Say, *under the table*."	Modeling
Child	"Table."	A wrong response
Clinician	Records the response as incorrect.	No corrective feedback
Clinician	"The car is under the hat. Where is the car? Say, *under the hat*."	Modeling
Child	"Under hat."	A correct response; omission of the article is ignored
Clinician	Records the response.	No verbal praise

Baserate at least 20 exemplars as shown on the next page.

Preposition *under* in Phrases

Exemplars and Baserate Recording Sheet

Print this page from the CD or photocopy this page for your clinical use.

The exemplars show the full sentence form, but the initial target for most children may be only the phrases ("under the   .")

Name/Age:		Date:
Goal: To establish the baserates of preposition *under* in phrases when asked questions while showing a picture or object.		Clinician:

Clinician's Comments:

Scoring: Correct: ✓   Incorrect or no response: X

Phrases with the preposition *under*	Evoked	Modeled
1. [The doll is] under the table.		
2. [The car is] under the hat.		
3. [The book is] under the chair.		
4. [The kitty is] under the bed.		
5. [The coin is] under the cup.		
6. [The girl is] under the tree.		
7. [The ball is] under the sofa.		
8. [The truck is] under the paper.		
9. [The crayon is] under the box.		
10. [The paper] is under the book.		
11. [The man is] under the umbrella.		
12. [The dog is] under the porch.		
13. [The soap is] under the sink.		
14. [The water is] under the bridge.		
15. [The flower is] under the leaf.		
16. [The grass is] under the basket.		
17. [The book is] under the light.		
18. [The boy is] under the roof.		
19. [The cat is] under the chair.		
20. [The snake] is under the stone.		
Percent correct baserate		

Replace or add exemplars as you see fit to suit an individual child. Consider the articles in the exemplars as optional. After establishing the baserates, initiate treatment. Use the protocols that follow.

Preposition *under* in Phrases

Treatment Protocols

At the beginning of each trial, have the child place a target object under another object (e.g., have the child place a doll under the table), or show a picture that represents the target phrase. Each time, point to the target object.

Scripts for Modeled Discrete Trial Training		Note
Clinician	"The doll is under the table. Where is the doll? Say, **under** the table."	Vocal emphasis on the target morpheme
Client	"Table."	A wrong response
Clinician	"No, that is not correct. Where is the doll? Say, **under** the table."	Corrective feedback; vocal emphasis on the target word
Client	"Under table." ["under the table."]	A correct response
Clinician	"Very good! You said **under** table!"	Verbal praise

Repeat the trials until the child gives 5 consecutively correct, imitated responses. When the child imitates 5 correct responses in sequence, fade the modeling. Always point to the target object before asking a question.

Scripts for Fading the Modeling		Note
Clinician	"The doll is under the table. Where is the doll? Say, *the doll is . . .*"	Partial modeling only
Client	"Table."	A wrong response
Clinician	"No, that is not correct. The doll is under the table. Where is the doll? Say, *the doll is . . .*"	Corrective feedback and partial modeling
Client	"Under table." ["Under the table."]	A correct response
Clinician	"Very good! You said *under table*!"	Verbal praise
Clinician	"Where is the doll?"	**An Evoked Trial**
Client	"Under table." ["Under the table."]	Correct answer

If the wrong responses persist on 4 to 5 evoked trials, reinstate partial or full modeling for a few trials, again fade the modeling, and re-present the evoked trials.

When the child meets the tentative learning criterion of 10 consecutively correct, nonimitated responses for a given exemplar, move on to the next exemplar. With this procedure, teach 6 to 8 exemplars. Use different exemplars as you see fit for a given child. Use the exemplars and the recording sheet given on the next page (or copy it from the CD).

Preposition *under* in Phrases

Exemplars and Treatment Recording Sheet

Print this page from the CD or photocopy this page for your clinical use.

Name/Age:	Date:
Goal: Production of the proposition *under* in phrases with 90% accuracy when asked questions while showing pictures.	Clinician:

Clinician's Comments:

Scoring: Correct: ✓   Incorrect or no response: X

Target skills	Discrete Trials														
	1	2	3	4	5	6	7	8	9	10	11	12	13	14	15
1. [The doll is] under the table.															
2. [The car is] under the hat.															
3. [The book is] under the chair.															
4. [The kitty is] under the bed.															
5. [The coin is] under the cup.															
6. [The girl is] under the tree.															
7. [The ball] is under the sofa.															
8. [The truck is] under the paper.															

Teach 6 to 8 exemplars each to a training criterion of 10 consecutively correct, nonimitated responses. Then, shift training to the sentence level. Baserate the production of the preposition in sentences before teaching.

Preposition *under* in Sentences

Baserate Protocols

At the beginning of each trial, either ask the child to place an object under something or show a relevant picture. Point to the object and then ask the specified question. Do not respond in any way to the child's correct, incorrect, or lack of responses.

Scripts for Evoked Baserate Trial		Note
Clinician	"Where is the doll?"	No modeling
Child	"Table." ["box"]	A wrong response
Clinician	Records the response as incorrect.	No corrective feedback
Clinician	"Where is the car?"	The next trial
Child	"Under hat." ["Under the hat."]	Scored as incorrect because the child did not produce the sentence
Clinician	Records the response as incorrect.	No corrective feedback

Administer the modeled baserate trials only after completing the evoked trials on all 20 (or more) exemplars. Again, let the child perform the required actions before starting each trial.

Scripts for Modeled Baserate Trial		Note
Clinician	"The doll is under the table. Where is the doll? Say, *the doll is under the table.*"	Modeling
Child	"Under table." ["Under the table."]	Scored as a wrong response
Clinician	Records the response as incorrect.	No corrective feedback
Clinician	"The car is under the hat. Where is the car? Say, *the car is under the hat.*"	Modeling
Child	"Car is under the hat."	A correct response; omission of the article is ignored
Clinician	Records the response.	No verbal praise

Baserate at least 20 exemplars as shown on the next page.

Preposition *under* in Sentences

Exemplars and Baserate Recording Sheet

Print this page from the CD or photocopy this page for your clinical use.

Name/Age:	Date:
Goal: To establish the baserates of the preposition *under* in sentences when asked questions while showing a picture or object.	Clinician:

Clinician's Comments:

Scoring: Correct: ✓   Incorrect or no response: X

Preposition *under* in Sentences	Evoked	Modeled
1. The doll is under the table.		
2. The car is under the hat.		
3. The book is under the chair.		
4. The kitty is under the bed.		
5. The coin is under the cup.		
6. The girl is under the tree.		
7. The ball is under the sofa.		
8. The truck is under the paper.		
9. The crayon is under the box.		
10. The paper is under the book.		
11. The man is under the umbrella.		
12. The dog is under the porch.		
13. The soap is under the sink.		
14. The water is under the bridge.		
15. The flower is under the leaf.		
16. The grass is under the basket.		
17. The book is under the light.		
18. The boy is under the roof.		
19. The cat is under the chair.		
20. The snake is under the stone.		
Percent correct baserate		

Replace or add new exemplars as you see fit for a given child.

After establishing the baserates for the target preposition in sentences, initiate treatment. Use the protocols given on the next page.

Preposition *under* in Sentences

Treatment Protocols

Teach 6 to 8 sentences with the preposition under *in sentences using the following script.*

Have the child perform the required action before starting treatment or show a relevant picture. Each time, point to the target objects.

Scripts for Modeled Discrete Trial Training		Note
Clinician	"The doll is under the table. Where is the doll? Say, ***the doll is under*** *the table*."	Vocal emphasis on the target words
Client	"Under table." ["Under the table."]	Scored as a wrong response
Clinician	"No, You didn't say the whole sentence. Where is the doll? Say, ***the doll is under*** *the table*."	Corrective feedback; vocal emphasis on the target words
Client	"The doll is under the table." ["Doll is under table."]	Scored as correct; one or more articles may be included
Clinician	"Very good! You said ***the doll is under*** *the table!*"	Verbal praise

Repeat the trials until the child gives 5 consecutively correct, imitated responses. When the child imitates 5 correct responses in sequence, fade the modeling. Always point to the target object before asking a question.

Scripts for Fading the Modeling		Note
Clinician	"The doll is under the table. Where is the doll? Say, *the doll is . . .* "	Partial modeling only
Client	"Table."	A wrong response
Clinician	"No, you didn't say the whole sentence. *The doll is under the table.* Where is the doll? Say, *the doll is . . .* "	Corrective feedback and partial modeling
Client	"The doll is under table." ["Doll is under the table."]	A correct response; optional article production
Clinician	"Very good! You said, *the doll is under table!*"	Verbal praise
Clinician	"Where is the doll?"	**An Evoked Trial**
Client	"The doll is under table." ["Doll is under the rug; The doll is under the table."]	Correct answer
Clinician	"Excellent! You said the whole sentence!"	Verbal praise

Preposition *under* in Sentences

Exemplars and Treatment Recording Sheet

Print this page from the CD or photocopy this page for your clinical use.

Name/Age:	Date:
Goal: Production of the proposition *under* in sentences with 90% accuracy when asked questions while showing pictures.	Clinician:

Clinician's Comments:

Scoring: Correct: ✓   Incorrect or no response: X

Target skills	Discrete Trials														
	1	2	3	4	5	6	7	8	9	10	11	12	13	14	15
1. The doll is under the table.															
2. The car is under the hat.															
3. The book is under the chair.															
4. The kitty is under the bed.															
5. The coin is under the cup.															
6. The girl is under the tree.															
7. The ball is under the sofa.															
8. The truck is under the paper.															

When the child has met the learning criterion of 10 consecutively correct, evoked (nonimitated) responses for each of the 6 to 8 target sentences, conduct a probe to see if the production of the preposition has generalized to previously baserated but untrained sentences.

Use the protocol given on the next page (or print it from the CD).

Preposition *under* in Sentences
Probe Protocols and Recording Sheet

Print this page from the CD or photocopy this page for your clinical use.

On the probes, present only the untrained exemplars (UT). When the child fails to meet the 90% correct probe criterion, either teach 2 to 4 new exemplars or give additional training trials on already trained exemplars. If needed, select new exemplars for probes. Probe at least 10 untrained exemplars. Alternate probes and treatment until the probe criterion is met.

Scripts for Probe Trials

Clinician	[Presents an untrained stimulus] "Where is the crayon?"	No modeling or prompts
Child	"The crayon is under the box."	A correct, generalized response
Clinician	Scores the response as correct.	Offers no reinforcement
Clinician	[Presents another untrained stimulus] "Where is the paper?"	The second probe trial
Child	"Under book."	A wrong probe response
Clinician	Scores the response as incorrect.	Offers no corrective feedback

Name:	Date:	Session #:
Age:	**Clinician:**	
Disorder: Language	**Target Behavior: Preposition *under* in Sentences (probe)**	
Untrained Stimuli	**Score: + correct; – incorrect or no responses**	
1. The crayon is under the box. (UT)		
2. The paper is under the book. (UT)		
3. The man is under the umbrella. (UT)		
4. The dog is under the porch. (UT)		
5. The soap is under the sink. (UT)		
6. The water is under the bridge. (UT)		
7. The flower is under the leaf. (UT)		
8. The grass is under the basket. (UT)		
9. The book is under the light. (UT)		
10. The boy is under the roof. (UT)		
11. The cat is under the chair. (UT)		
12. The snake is under the stone. (UT)		
Percent correct probe (Criterion: 90%)		

If the child does not meet the probe criterion, give additional training on already trained sentences and subsequently readminister the probe trials. When the child meets the 90% correct probe criterion for the preposition under in sentences, shift training to other morphologic features (such as the preposition behind as shown next) or to conversational speech in which the preposition under is monitored and reinforced.

Preposition *behind*
Preposition *behind* in Phrases
Baserate Protocols

When practical, help the child perform the required action. For instance, have the child place a toy cat behind a small box placed on the desk. Let the object that lies behind something be visible to the child throughout the teaching session. Point to the object. When this is not possible, use realistic pictures and point to the object or person behind something before asking the relevant question.

Administer the evoked trials first followed by modeled trials. Do not provide feedback on any trials; just record the child's responses on the recording sheet provided on the next page or printed from the CD.

Note: *The target phrases include the definite article. The clinician models the phrase with the article, but does not emphasize it or provide contingent consequences (reinforcement or corrective feedback) for it. A child may or may not produce the article. Score the responses solely on the basis of presence or absence of the preposition. Do not score it incorrect if the child fails to produce the article as it is not the target in this segment of teaching.*

Scripts for Evoked Baserate Trial		Note
Clinician	[after the child has placed a toy cat behind a box] "Where is the cat?"	No modeling
Child	"Box."	A wrong response
Clinician	Records the response as incorrect.	No corrective feedback
Clinician	[after the child has placed an apple behind a bag] "Where is the apple?"	The next trial
Child	"Behind bag."	A correct response; the omission of the article is ignored
Clinician	Records the response as correct.	No verbal praise

Administer the modeled baserate trials only after completing the evoked trials on all 20 (or more) exemplars. Again, let the child perform the required actions before starting each trial.

Scripts for Modeled Baserate Trial		Note
Clinician	"The cat is behind the box. Where is the cat? Say, *behind the box.*"	Modeling
Child	"Box."	A wrong response
Clinician	Records the response as incorrect.	No corrective feedback
Clinician	"The apple is behind the bag. Where is the apple? Say, *behind the bag.*"	Modeling
Child	"Behind bag."	A correct response; omission of the article is ignored
Clinician	Records the response.	No verbal praise

Baserate at least 20 exemplars as shown on the next page.

Preposition *behind* in Phrases

Exemplars and Baserate Recording Sheet

Print this page from the CD or photocopy this page for your clinical use.

The exemplars show the full sentence form, but the initial target for most children may be only the phrases ("behind the ____"). The noun phrase within the brackets is optional at this level of training.

Replace or add exemplars as you see fit to suit an individual child.

Name/Age:	Date:
Goal: To establish the baserates of the preposition *behind* in phrases when asked questions while showing a picture or object.	Clinician:

Clinician's Comments:

Scoring: Correct: ✓   Incorrect or no response: X

Sentence Level	Evoked	Modeled
1. [The cat is] behind the box.		
2. [The apple is] behind the bag.		
3. [The balloon is] behind the chair.		
4. [The book is] behind the ball.		
5. [The car is] behind the bus.		
6. [The cup is] behind the pot.		
7. [The pencil is] behind the book.		
8. [The key is] behind the purse.		
9. [The man is] behind the tree.		
10. [The teacher is] behind the desk.		
11. [The bike is] behind the house.		
12. [The girl is] behind the chair.		
13. [The dog is] behind the fence.		
14. [The sun is] behind the clouds.		
15. [The bird is] behind the nest.		
16. [The ball is] behind the TV.		
17. [The frog is] behind the rock.		
18. [The lion is] behind the bushes.		
19. [The woman is] behind the door.		
20. [The house is] behind the hill.		
Percent correct baserate		

After establishing the baserates, initiate treatment. Use the protocols given on the next page.

Preposition *behind* in Phrases

Treatment Protocols

At the beginning of each trial, have the child place a target object behind another object (e.g., have the child place a toy cat behind a box) or show a picture that represents the target phrase. Each time, point to the target object.

Scripts for Modeled Discrete Trial Training		Note
Clinician	"The cat is behind the box. Where is the cat? Say, **behind** the box."	Vocal emphasis on the target morpheme
Child	"Box."	A wrong response
Clinician	"No, that is not correct. Where is the cat? Say, **behind** the box."	Corrective feedback; vocal emphasis on the target word
Child	"Behind box." ["Behind the box."]	A correct response
Clinician	"Very good! You said **behind** the box!"	Verbal praise

Repeat the trials until the child gives 5 consecutively correct, imitated responses. When the child imitates 5 correct responses in sequence, fade the modeling. Always point to the target object before asking a question.

Scripts for Fading the Modeling		Note
Clinician	"The cat is behind the box. Where is the cat? Say, *the cat is . . .*"	Partial modeling only
Child	"Behind." ["Box."]	A wrong response
Clinician	"No, that is not correct. The cat is behind the box. Where is the cat? Say, *the cat is . . .*"	Corrective feedback and partial modeling
Child	"Behind box." ["Behind the box."]	A correct response
Clinician	"Very good! You said *behind box*!"	Verbal praise
Clinician	"Where is the cat?"	**An Evoked Trial**
Child	"Behind box." ["Behind the box."]	Correct answer

If the wrong responses persist on 4 to 5 evoked trials, reinstate partial or full modeling for a few trials, again fade the modeling, and re-present the evoked trials.

When the child meets the tentative learning criterion of 10 consecutively correct, nonimitated responses for a given exemplar, move on to the next exemplar. With this procedure, teach 6 to 8 exemplars. Use different exemplars as you see fit for a given child. Use the exemplars and the recording sheet given on the next page (or print it from the CD).

Preposition *behind* in Phrases

Exemplars and Treatment Recording Sheet

Print this page from the CD or photocopy this page for your clinical use.

Name/Age:	Date:
Goal: Production of the proposition *behind* in phrases with 90% accuracy when asked questions while showing pictures.	Clinician:

Clinician's Comments:

Scoring: Correct: ✓   Incorrect or no response: X

Target skills	Discrete Trials														
	1	2	3	4	5	6	7	8	9	10	11	12	13	14	15
1. [The cat is] behind the box.															
2. [The apple is] behind the bag.															
3. [The balloon is] behind the chair.															
4. [The book is] behind the ball.															
5. [The car is] behind the bus.															
6. [The cup is] behind the pot.															
7. [The pencil is] behind the book.															
8. [The key is] behind the purse.															

Teach 6 to 8 exemplars each to a training criterion of 10 consecutively correct nonimitated responses. Then, shift training to the sentence level. Baserate the production of the preposition in sentences before initiating treatment.

Preposition *behind* in Sentences

Baserate Protocols

At the beginning of each trial, either ask the child to place an object behind something or show a relevant picture. Point to the object and then ask the specified question. Do not respond in any way to the child's correct, incorrect, or lack of responses.

Scripts for Evoked Baserate Trial		Note
Clinician	"Where is the cat?"	No modeling
Child	"Box." ["box"]	A wrong response
Clinician	Records the response as incorrect.	No corrective feedback
Clinician	"Where is the apple?"	The next trial
Child	"Behind bag." ["Behind the bag."]	Scored as incorrect because the child did not produce the sentence.
Clinician	Records the response as incorrect.	No corrective feedback

Administer the modeled baserate trials only after completing the evoked trials on all 20 (or more) exemplars. Again, let the child perform the required actions before starting each trial.

Scripts for Modeled Baserate Trial		Note
Clinician	"The cat is behind the box. Where is the cat? Say, *the cat is behind the box.*"	Modeling
Child	"Behind box." ["Behind the box."]	Scored as a wrong response
Clinician	Records the response as incorrect.	No corrective feedback
Clinician	"The apple is behind the bag. Where is the apple? Say, *the apple is behind the bag.*"	Modeling
Child	"Apple is behind the bag."	A correct response; omission of the article is ignored
Clinician	Records the response.	No verbal praise

Baserate at least 20 exemplars as shown on the next page.

Preposition *behind* in Sentences

Exemplars and Baserate Recording Sheet

Print this page from the CD or photocopy this page for your clinical use.

Name/Age:	Date:
Goal: To establish the baserates of the preposition *behind* in sentences when asked questions while showing a picture or object.	Clinician:

Clinician's Comments:

Scoring: Correct: ✓   Incorrect or no response: X

Preposition *behind* in Sentences	Evoked	Modeled
1. The cat is behind the box.		
2. The apple is behind the bag.		
3. The balloon is behind the chair.		
4. The book is behind the ball.		
5. The car is behind the bus.		
6. The cup is behind the pot.		
7. The pencil is behind the book.		
8. The key is behind the purse.		
9. The man is behind the tree.		
10. The teacher is behind the desk.		
11. The bike is behind the house.		
12. The girl is behind the chair.		
13. The dog is behind the fence.		
14. The sun is behind the clouds.		
15. The bird is behind the nest.		
16. The ball is behind the TV.		
17. The frog is behind the rock.		
18. The lion is behind the bushes.		
19. The woman is behind the door.		
20. The house is behind the hill.		
Percent correct baserate		

Replace or add new exemplars as you see fit for a given child.

After establishing the baserates for the target preposition in sentences, initiate treatment. Use the protocols given on the next page.

Preposition *behind* in Sentences

Treatment Protocols

Teach 6 to 8 sentences with the preposition behind *in sentences using the following script.*

Have the child perform the required action before starting treatment or show a relevant picture. Each time, point to the target objects.

Scripts for Modeled Discrete Trial Training		Note
Clinician	"The cat is behind the box. Where is the cat? Say, **the cat is behind** the box."	Vocal emphasis on the target words
Child	"Behind box." ["Behind the box."]	Scored as a wrong response
Clinician	"No, You didn't say the whole sentence. Where is the cat? Say, **the cat is behind** the box."	Corrective feedback; vocal emphasis on the target words
Child	"The cat is behind the box." ["Cat is behind box."]	Scored as correct; one or more article may be included
Clinician	"Very good! You said **the cat is behind the box**!"	Verbal praise

Repeat the trials until the child gives 5 consecutively correct, imitated responses. When the child imitates 5 correct responses in sequence, fade the modeling. Always point to the target object before asking a question.

Scripts for Fading the Modeling		Note
Clinician	"The cat is behind the box. Where is the cat? Say, the *cat is . . .*"	Partial modeling only
Child	"Box."	A wrong response
Clinician	"No, you didn't say the whole sentence. *The cat is behind the box.* Where is the cat? Say, *the cat is . . .*"	Corrective feedback and partial modeling
Child	"The cat is behind box." ["Cat is behind the box."]	A correct response; optional article production
Clinician	"Very good! You said, *the cat is behind box*!"	Verbal praise
Clinician	"Where is the cat?"	**An Evoked Trial**
Child	"The cat is behind box." ["Cat is behind the box"; "The cat is behind the box."]	Correct answer
Clinician	"Excellent! You said the whole sentence!"	Verbal praise

Preposition *behind* in Sentences

Exemplars and Treatment Recording Sheet

Print this page from the CD or photocopy this page for your clinical use.

Name/Age:	Date:
Goal: Production of the proposition *behind* in sentences with 90% accuracy when asked questions while showing pictures.	Clinician:

Clinician's Comments:

Scoring: Correct: ✓   Incorrect or no response: X

Target skills	Discrete Trials														
	1	2	3	4	5	6	7	8	9	10	11	12	13	14	15
1. The cat is behind the box.															
2. The apple is behind the bag.															
3. The balloon is behind the chair.															
4. The book is behind the ball.															
5. The car is behind the bus.															
6. The cup is behind the pot.															
7. The pencil is behind the book.															
8. The key is behind the purse.															

When the child has met the learning criterion of 10 consecutively correct, evoked (nonimitated) responses for each of the 6 to 8 target sentences, conduct a probe to see if the production of the preposition has generalized to previously baserated but untrained sentences.

Use the protocols given on the next page (or print it from the CD).

Preposition *behind* in Sentences

Probe Protocols and Recording Sheet

Print this page from the CD or photocopy this page for your clinical use.

On the probes, present only the untrained exemplars (UT). When the child fails to meet the 90% correct probe criterion, either teach 2 to 4 new exemplars or give additional training trials on already trained exemplars. If needed, select new exemplars for probes. Probe at least 10 untrained exemplars. Alternate probes and treatment until the probe criterion is met.

Scripts for Probe Trials

Clinician	[Presents an untrained stimulus] "Where is the man?"	No modeling or prompts
Child	"The man is behind the tree."	A correct, generalized response
Clinician	Scores the response as correct.	Offers no reinforcement
Clinician	[Presents another untrained stimulus] "Where is the teacher?"	The second probe trial
Child	"Behind desk."	A wrong probe response
Clinician	Scores the response as incorrect.	Offers no corrective feedback

Name:	Date:	Session #:
Age:	**Clinician:**	
Disorder: Language	**Target Behavior: Preposition *behind* in Sentences (probe)**	
Untrained Stimuli	**Score: + correct; – incorrect or no responses**	
1. The man is behind the tree. (UT)		
2. The teacher is behind the desk. (UT)		
3. The bike is behind the house. (UT)		
4. The girl is behind the chair. (UT)		
5. The dog is behind the fence. (UT)		
6. The sun is behind the clouds. (UT)		
7. The bird is behind the nest. (UT)		
8. The ball is behind the TV. (UT)		
9. The frog is behind the rock. (UT)		
10. The lion is behind the bushes. (UT)		
11. The woman is behind the door. (UT)		
12. The house is behind the hill. (UT)		
Percent correct probe (Criterion: 90%)		

If the child does not meet the probe criterion, give additional training on already trained sentences and subsequently readminister the probe trials. When the child meets the 90% correct sentence probe criterion for the preposition behind, *shift training to other morphologic features or to conversational speech in which the preposition* behind *is monitored and reinforced.*

Present Progressive *ing*

Overview

Present progressive *ing* is a grammatic morpheme that children master early. The three children in Brown's longitudinal study (1973) mastered this morpheme before any other. The present progressive *ing* is important for building sentences and for expanding the language skills in children. A variety of sentences require the present progressive. Most importantly, the present progressive is essential in sentences that combine nouns and verbs.

Children with language disorders typically fail to learn this essential morpheme. Therefore, it is an important functional treatment target for children with language disorders.

General Training Strategy

In teaching the present progressive *ing*, clinicians often use pictures to depict the actions of animate nouns (people and animals). Clinicians may more effectively use various toys to demonstrate miniature actions to evoke phrases and sentences with the present progressive. Such actions may hold the child's interest better than the pictures. Nonetheless, pictures are essential to teach a broad range of sentences with the present progressive because many actions are not readily and realistically demonstrated in the clinic.

The present progressive is best taught first in words. It does not lend itself to teaching in phrases. Therefore, when the child masters a few exemplars in single words, the clinician should move on to teaching the morpheme in short and simple sentences.

Present Progressive *ing* in Words

Baserate Protocols

Demonstrate a miniature action or show a relevant picture before starting each trial. For instance, you can hold a toy bird and simulate its flying action. When using pictures, point to the action (e.g., cooking or running).

Administer the evoked trials first followed by modeled trials. Do not provide feedback on any trials; just record the responses on the recording sheet provided on the next page or printed from the CD.

Note that the target phrases include the definite article and the auxiliary is. *The clinician models the phrase with the article and the auxiliary, but does not emphasize them or provide contingent consequences (reinforcement or corrective feedback) while teaching the present progressive* ing. *A child may or may not produce the article or the auxiliary. Score the responses solely on the basis of presence or absence of the present progressive. Do not score it incorrect if the child fails to produce the article or the auxiliary as they are not the target in this segment of teaching.*

Alternatively, the clinician may emphasize both the auxiliary is *and the* ing *to teach both at the same time. If this is the clinician's choice, the reinforcement would depend on the production of both the targets. The article would still be an optional feature.*

Scripts for Evoked Baserate Trial		Note
Clinician	[showing the picture of a man cooking] "What is the man doing?"	No modeling
Child	"Cook."	A wrong response
Clinician	Records the response as incorrect.	No corrective feedback
Clinician	[showing the picture of a smiling baby] "What is the baby doing?"	The next trial
Child	"Smiling."	A correct response
Clinician	Records the response as correct.	No verbal praise

Administer the modeled baserate trials only after completing the evoked trials on all 20 (or more) exemplars. Again, let the child perform the required actions before starting each trial.

Scripts for Modeled Baserate Trial		Note
Clinician	"The man is cooking. What is the man doing? Say, *cooking*."	Modeling
Child	"Man cook." ["Cook."]	A wrong response
Clinician	Records the response as incorrect.	No corrective feedback
Clinician	"The baby is smiling. What is the baby doing? Say, *smiling*."	Modeling
Child	"Smiling."	A correct response
Clinician	Records the response.	No verbal praise

Baserate at least 20 exemplars as shown on the next page.

Present Progressive *ing* in Words

Exemplars and Baserate Recording Sheet

Print this page from the CD or photocopy this page for your clinical use.

Replace or add exemplars as you see fit to suit an individual child.

Name/Age:	Date:
Goal: To establish the baserates of the present progressive *ing* in words when asked questions while showing a picture or object.	Clinician:

Clinician's Comments:

Scoring: Correct: ✓   Incorrect or no response: X

Words with *ing*	Evoked	Modeled
1. [The man is] cooking.		
2. [The baby is] smiling.		
3. [The girl is] dancing.		
4. [The boy is] swimming.		
5. [The dog is] drinking.		
6. [The man is] eating.		
7. [The bird is] feeding.		
8. [The frog is] jumping.		
9. [The clown is] laughing.		
10. [The man is] mowing.		
11. [The girl is] playing.		
12. [The woman is] pouring.		
13. [The lion is] running.		
14. [The man is] shaving.		
15. [The bird is] flying.		
16. [The cat is] sitting.		
17. [The woman is] sleeping.		
18. [The girl is] reading.		
19. [The boy is] walking.		
20. [The woman is] writing.		
Percent correct baserate		

Note: *The noun phrases in brackets are optional when teaching the verb + ing. Use the following protocols to teach the present progressive in words.*

Present Progressive *ing* in Words

Treatment Protocols

At the beginning of each trial, have the child perform a miniature action or place an action picture in front of the child.

Scripts for Modeled Discrete Trial Training		Note
Clinician	"The man is cooking. What is the man doing? Say, cook**ing**."	Vocal emphasis on the target morpheme
Child	"Cook."	A wrong response
Clinician	"No, that is not correct. What is the man doing? Say, cook**ing**."	Corrective feedback; vocal emphasis on the *ing*
Child	"Cooking."	A correct response
Clinician	"Very good! You said cook**ing**!"	Verbal praise

Repeat the trials until the child gives 5 consecutively correct, imitated responses. When the child imitates 5 correct responses in sequence, fade the modeling. Always point to the target object before asking a question.

Scripts for Fading the Modeling		Note
Clinician	"The man is cooking. What is the man doing? Say, *coo . . .*"	Partial modeling only
Child	"Cook."	A wrong response
Clinician	"No, that is not correct. The man is cooking. What is the man doing? Say, *coo . . .*"	Corrective feedback and partial modeling
Child	"Cooking."	A correct response
Clinician	"Very good! You said *cooking*!"	Verbal praise
Clinician	"What is the man doing?"	**An Evoked Trial**
Child	"Cooking." ["Man cooking."]	Correct answer

If the wrong responses persist on 4 to 5 evoked trials, reinstate partial or full modeling for a few trials, again fade the modeling, and re-present the evoked trials.

When the child meets the tentative learning criterion of 10 consecutively correct, nonimitated responses for a given exemplar, move on to the next exemplar. With this procedure, teach 6 to 8 exemplars. Use different exemplars as you see fit for a given child. Use the exemplars and the recording sheet given on the next page (or copy it from the CD).

Present Progressive *ing* in Words

Exemplars and Treatment Recording Sheet

Print this page from the CD or photocopy this page for your clinical use.

Name/Age:	Date:
Goal: Production of the present progressive *ing* in words with 90% accuracy when asked questions while showing pictures.	Clinician:

Clinician's Comments:

Scoring: Correct: ✓   Incorrect or no response: X

Target skills	Discrete Trials														
	1	2	3	4	5	6	7	8	9	10	11	12	13	14	15
1. [The man is] cooking.															
2. [The baby is] smiling.															
3. [The girl is] dancing.															
4. [The boy is] swimming.															
5. [The dog is] drinking.															
6. [The man is] eating.															
7. [The bird is] feeding.															
8. [The frog is jumping.]															

Teach 6 to 8 exemplars each to a training criterion of 10 consecutively correct nonimitated responses. Then, shift training to the sentence level. Before teaching the ing *in sentences, baserate their productions. Use the protocols that follow.*

Present Progressive *ing* in Sentences

Baserate Protocols

At the beginning of each trial, either demonstrate a miniature action or show a relevant picture. Do not respond in any way to the child's correct, incorrect, or lack of responses.

Scripts for Evoked Baserate Trial		Note
Clinician	"What is the man doing? Start with, *the man . . .*"	Prompting the full sentence
Child	"Cook."	A wrong response
Clinician	Records the response as incorrect.	No corrective feedback
Clinician	"What is the baby doing? Start with, *the baby . . .*"	The next trial
Child	"Baby smiling." [No response]	Scored as incorrect because the child did not produce the sentence
Clinician	Records the response as incorrect.	No corrective feedback

Administer the modeled baserate trials only after completing the evoked trials on all 20 (or more) exemplars. Again, let the child perform the required actions before starting each trial.

Scripts for Modeled Baserate Trial		Note
Clinician	"The man is cooking. What is the man doing? Say, *the man is cooking.*"	Modeling
Child	"Man cook."	Scored as a wrong response
Clinician	Records the response as incorrect.	No corrective feedback
Clinician	"The baby is smiling. What is the baby doing? Say, *the baby is smiling.*"	Modeling
Child	"Baby is smiling."	A correct response; omission of the article is ignored
Clinician	Records the response.	No verbal praise

Baserate at least 20 exemplars as shown on the next page.

Present Progressive *ing* in Sentences

Exemplars and Baserate Recording Sheet

Print this page from the CD or photocopy this page for your clinical use.

Name/Age:	Date:
Goal: To establish the baserates of the present progressive *ing* in sentences when asked questions while showing a picture or object.	Clinician:

Clinician's Comments:

Scoring: Correct: ✓   Incorrect or no response: X

Sentences with *ing*	Evoked	Modeled
1. The man is cooking.		
2. The baby is smiling.		
3. The girl is dancing.		
4. The boy is swimming.		
5. The dog is drinking.		
6. The man is eating.		
7. The bird is feeding.		
8. The frog is jumping.		
9. The clown is laughing.		
10. The man is mowing.		
11. The girl is playing.		
12. The woman is pouring.		
13. The lion is running.		
14. The man is shaving.		
15. The bird is flying.		
16. The cat is sitting.		
17. The woman is sleeping.		
18. The girl is reading.		
19. The boy is walking.		
20. The woman is writing.		
Percent correct baserate		

Replace or add new exemplars as you see fit for a given child.

After establishing the baserates for the present progressive in sentences, initiate treatment. Use the protocols given on the next page.

PRESENT PROGRESSIVE *ING*   **151**

Present Progressive *ing* in Sentences

Treatment Protocols

Teach 6 to 8 sentences with the present progressive ing *in sentences using the following script.*

Show a relevant picture before you ask the question. Each time, point to the target objects.

Scripts for Modeled Discrete Trial Training		Note
Clinician	"The man is cooking. What is the man doing? Say, **the man is cooking**."	Vocal emphasis on the target words
Child	"Man cook."	Scored as a wrong response
Clinician	"No, You didn't say the whole sentence. What is the man doing? Say, **the man is cooking**."	Corrective feedback; vocal emphasis on the target words
Child	"The man is cooking." ["Man is cooking."]	Scored as correct; the article may be omitted
Clinician	"Very good! You said, **the man is cooking**!"	Verbal praise

Repeat the trials until the child gives 5 consecutively correct, imitated responses. When the child imitates 5 correct responses in sequence, fade the modeling. Always point to the target object before asking a question.

Scripts for Fading the Modeling		Note
Clinician	"The man is cooking. What is the man doing? Say, the *man is* . . ."	Partial modeling only
Child	"Cooking."	A wrong response
Clinician	"No, you didn't say the whole sentence. *The man is cooking.* What is the man doing? Say, *the man is* . . ."	Corrective feedback and partial modeling
Child	"The man is cooking." ["Man is cooking."]	A correct response; optional article production
Clinician	"Very good! You said, *the man is cooking*!"	Verbal praise
Clinician	"What is the man doing?"	**An Evoked Trial**
Child	"The man is cooking." ["Man is cooking."]	Correct answer
Clinician	"Excellent! You said the whole sentence!"	Verbal praise

Present Progressive *ing* in Sentences

Exemplars and Treatment Recording Sheet

Print this page from the CD or photocopy this page for your clinical use.

Name/Age:	Date:
Goal: Production of the present progressive *ing* in sentences with 90% accuracy when asked questions while showing pictures.	Clinician:

Clinician's Comments:

Scoring: Correct: ✓   Incorrect or no response: X

Target skills	Discrete Trials														
	1	2	3	4	5	6	7	8	9	10	11	12	13	14	15
1. The man is cooking.															
2. The baby is smiling.															
3. The girl is dancing.															
4. The boy is swimming.															
5. The dog is drinking.															
6. The man is eating.															
7. The bird is feeding.															
8. The frog is jumping.															

When the child has met the learning criterion of 10 consecutively correct, evoked (nonimitated) responses for each of the 6 to 8 target sentences, conduct a probe to see if the production of ing has generalized to previously baserated but untrained sentences.

Use the protocol given on the next page (or print it from the CD).

Present Progressive *ing* in Sentences
Probe Protocols and Recording Sheet

Print this page from the CD or photocopy this page for your clinical use.

On the probes, present only the untrained exemplars (UT). When the child fails to meet the 90% correct probe criterion, either teach 2 to 4 new exemplars or give additional training trials on already trained exemplars. If needed, select new exemplars for probes. Probe at least 10 untrained exemplars. Alternate probes and treatment until the probe criterion is met.

Scripts for Probe Trials

Clinician	[Presents an untrained stimulus] "What is the clown doing?"	No modeling or prompts.
Child	"The clown is laughing."	A correct, generalized response
Clinician	Scores the response as correct.	Offers no reinforcement
Clinician	[Presents another untrained stimulus] "What is the man doing?"	The second probe trial
Child	"Mow."	A wrong probe response
Clinician	Scores the response as incorrect.	Offers no corrective feedback

Name:	Date:	Session #:
Age:	**Clinician:**	
Disorder: Language	**Target: Present Progressive *ing* in Sentences (probe)**	
Untrained Stimuli	**Score: + correct; − incorrect or no responses**	
1. The clown is laughing.		
2. The man is mowing.		
3. The girl is playing.		
4. The woman is pouring.		
5. The lion is running.		
6. The man is shaving.		
7. The bird is flying.		
8. The cat is sitting.		
9. The woman is sleeping.		
10. The girl is reading.		
11. The boy is walking.		
12. The woman is writing.		
Percent correct probe (Criterion: 90%)		

If the child does not meet the probe criterion, give additional training on already trained sentences and subsequently readminister the probe trials. When the child meets the 90% correct sentence probe criterion for the present progressive, shift training to other morphologic features or to conversational speech in which the target skills are monitored and reinforced.

Auxiliaries and Copulas

Overview

The English auxiliary system is essential for expanding sentences and to express actions or inherent qualities of persons or objects. Linguists distinguish auxiliaries from copulas because they serve different grammatical functions. For instance, auxiliaries (e.g., *is*) are necessary in sentences that contain main verbs (e.g., *walking: he is walking*). Copulas, on the other hand, are necessary in sentences that include adjectives (e.g., *nice* as in *she is nice*). Note that an auxiliary and a copula take the same form (and are spelled the same), but their grammatical functions are different.

There are various forms of auxiliary and copula. The most common are the singular and plural forms (e.g., *is* and *are*), the present and the past tense forms (e.g., *is* and *was*), and the contractible (e.g., *he's* for *he is* and *she's* for *she is*) and the uncontractible forms (e.g., as in *he was* and *you were*). Because each auxiliary and copula has these variations, the clinician should set aside sufficient time to teaching them. Clinical judgment is that it is sufficient to teach the uncontracted forms (e.g., *she is* instead of *she's*; *Mommy is* instead of *Mommy's*) of auxiliary or copula. The child who learns to produce the auxiliary and copula in uncontracted forms correctly, may communicate effectively, even if the contracted forms are not used.

General Training Strategy

Children may master certain forms of copula before they master forms of auxiliary (Brown, 1973). Therefore, some clinicians believe that copula should be taught before auxiliary. However, clinical research has demonstrated that the basic distinction between the auxiliary and copula is not relevant for teaching children who do not produce them. Treatment research has shown that the theoretical distinction between the two does not hold in empirical teaching (Hegde, 1980; Hegde & McConn, 1981; Hegde, Noll, & Pecora, 1979). This means that the auxiliary and the copula belong to a single response class. Teaching one will result in generalized production of the other. Therefore, the clinician should not be concerned about which one to teach first. Teaching either one will usually be sufficient. Probes, however, are necessary to confirm this. When the auxiliary is taught, the clinician should probe for copular productions and vice versa. If there is no generalized production of the untrained feature, the clinician can then teach it.

Auxiliary *is*
Auxiliary *is* in Basic Sentences
Baserate Protocols

Note: *If you already have taught the* **present progressive ing in sentences**, *the child may have mastered the auxiliary form used in those sentences. It is possible that you may teach the auxiliary before the present progressive ing; in which case, the child who learns the auxiliary will have mastered the present progressive ing. Protocols are given for both the present progressives and auxiliaries so the clinician can teach either form first. Baserating the other form will then help decide whether it is necessary to teach it.*

Teach auxiliaries as you would the present progressive. Demonstrate a miniature action or show a relevant picture before starting each trial. For instance, you can hold a toy horse and simulate its running action. When using pictures, point to the action (e.g., cooking or running).

Note that the target sentences include the definite article. The clinician models the phrase with the article, but does not emphasize it or make reinforcement contingent on it while teaching the auxiliary. A child may or may not produce the article. Score the responses solely on the basis of presence or absence of the auxiliary.

Alternatively, the clinician may emphasize both the auxiliary and the article to teach them simultaneously. If this is the clinician's choice, the reinforcement would depend on the production of both targets.

Scripts for Evoked Baserate Trial		Note
Clinician	[showing the picture of a girl writing] "What is the girl doing?"	No modeling
Child	"Girl write." ["Write."]	A wrong response
Clinician	Records the response as incorrect.	No corrective feedback
Clinician	[showing the picture of a woman walking] "What is the woman doing?"	The next trial
Child	"Woman is walking."	A correct response
Clinician	Records the response as correct.	No verbal praise

Administer the modeled baserate trials only after completing the evoked trials on all 20 (or more) exemplars.

Scripts for Modeled Baserate Trial		Note
Clinician	"The girl is writing. What is the girl doing? Say, *the girl is writing*."	Modeling
Child	"Girl write." ["girl is writing."]	A wrong response
Clinician	Records the response as incorrect.	No corrective feedback
Clinician	"The woman is walking. What is the woman doing? Say, *the woman is walking*."	Modeling
Child	"The woman is walking."	A correct response
Clinician	Records the response.	No verbal praise

Baserate at least 20 exemplars as shown on the next page.

Auxiliary *is* in Basic Sentences

Exemplars and Baserate Recording Sheet

Print this page from the CD or photocopy this page for your clinical use.

Replace or add exemplars as you see fit to suit an individual child.

Name/Age:	Date:
Goal: To establish the baserates of the auxiliary *is* in basic sentences when asked questions while showing a picture or demonstrating an action.	Clinician:

Clinician's Comments:

Scoring: Correct: ✓   Incorrect or no response: X

Auxiliary *is* in Basic Sentences	Evoked	Modeled
1. [The] girl is writing.		
2. [The] woman is walking.		
3. [The] girl is eating.		
4. [The] woman is reading.		
5. [The] girl is buying.		
6. [The] woman is kicking.		
7. [The] girl is talking.		
8. [The] woman is digging.		
9. [The] boy is sitting.		
10. [The] man is cutting.		
11. [The] boy is opening.		
12. [The] man is cooking.		
13. [The] boy is building.		
14. [The] man is sleeping.		
15. [The] boy is throwing.		
16. [The] man is riding.		
17. [The] bug is moving.		
18. [The] deer is running.		
19. The] cat is eating.		
20. [The] dog is going.		
Percent correct baserate		

Note: *Unless the child has already been taught or has been producing it without teaching, the definite article shown in brackets is optional when teaching the auxiliary.*

After establishing the baserates, initiate treatment. Use the protocols that follow.

Auxiliary *is* in Basic Sentences

Treatment Protocol

At the beginning of each trial, have the child perform a miniature action or place an action picture in front of the child.

Scripts for Modeled Discrete Trial Training		Note
Clinician	"The girl is writing. What is the girl doing? Say, *the girl **is** writing*."	Vocal emphasis on the target morpheme
Child	"Writing." ["Girl writing."]	A wrong response
Clinician	"No, that is not correct. What is the girl doing? Say, *the girl **is** writing*."	Corrective feedback; vocal emphasis on the *is*
Child	"Girl is writing." ["The girl is writing."]	A correct response
Clinician	"Very good! You said the girl **is** writing!"	Verbal praise

Repeat the trials until the child gives 5 consecutively correct, imitated responses. When the child imitates 5 correct responses in sequence, fade the modeling. Always point to the action picture or perform a miniature action before asking a question.

Scripts for Fading the Modeling		Note
Clinician	"The girl is writing. What is the girl doing? Say, *the girl . . .*"	Partial modeling only
Child	"Write."	A wrong response
Clinician	"No, that is not correct. The girl is writing. What is the girl doing? Say, *the girl . . .*"	Corrective feedback and partial modeling
Child	"The girl is writing." ["Girl is writing."]	A correct response
Clinician	"Very good! You said, *the girl is writing*!"	Verbal praise
Clinician	"What is the girl doing?"	**An Evoked Trial**
Child	"The girl is writing." ["Girl is writing."]	Correct answer

If the wrong responses persist on 4 to 5 evoked trials, reinstate partial or full modeling for a few trials, again fade the modeling, and re-present the evoked trials.

When the child meets the tentative learning criterion of 10 consecutively correct, nonimitated responses for a given exemplar, move on to the next exemplar. With this procedure, teach 8 to 10 exemplars. Use different exemplars as you see fit for a given child. Use the exemplars and the recording sheet on the next page (or copy it from the CD).

Auxiliary *is* in Basic Sentences

Exemplars and Treatment Recording Sheet

Print this page from the CD or photocopy this page for your clinical use.

Name/Age:	Date:
Goal: Production of the auxiliary *is* in basic sentences with 90% accuracy when asked questions while showing pictures or demonstrating actions.	Clinician:

Clinician's Comments:

Scoring: Correct: ✓   Incorrect or no response: X

Target skills	Discrete Trials														
	1	2	3	4	5	6	7	8	9	10	11	12	13	14	15
1. [The] girl is writing.															
2. [The] woman is walking.															
3. [The] girl is eating.															
4. [The] woman is reading.															
5. [The] girl is buying.															
6. [The] woman is kicking.															
7. [The] girl is talking.															
8. [The] woman is digging.															
9. [The] boy is sitting.															
10. [The] man is cutting.															

Teach 8 to 10 basic sentence exemplars each to a training criterion of 10 consecutively correct non-imitated responses. Then, shift training to the expanded sentence level. Before teaching the auxiliary in expanded sentences, baserate their productions. Use the protocols that follow.

Auxiliary *is* in Expanded Sentences

Baserate Protocols

At the beginning of each trial, either demonstrate a miniature action or show a relevant picture. Do not respond in any way to the child's correct, incorrect, or lack of responses.

Scripts for Evoked Baserate Trial		**Note**
Clinician	[showing the picture of a girl writing] "The girl is writing a letter. What is the girl doing?"	The new target response is pointed out
Child	"Girl write." ["Write."]	A wrong response
Clinician	Records the response as incorrect.	No corrective feedback
Clinician	[showing the picture of a woman walking] "The woman is walking to her house. What is the woman doing?"	The next trial
Child	"Woman is walking to her house."	A correct response
Clinician	Records the response as correct.	No verbal praise

Administer the modeled baserate trials only after completing the evoked trials on all 20 (or more) exemplars.

Scripts for Modeled Baserate Trial		**Note**
Clinician	"The girl is writing a letter. What is the girl doing? Say, *the girl is writing a letter.*"	Modeling
Child	"Girl writing." ["Girl is writing."]	A wrong response
Clinician	Records the response as incorrect.	No corrective feedback
Clinician	"The woman is walking to her house. What is the woman doing? Say, *the woman is walking to her house.*"	Modeling
Child	"The woman is walking to her house."	A correct response
Clinician	Records the response.	No verbal praise

Baserate at least 20 exemplars as shown on the next page.

Auxiliary *is* in Expanded Sentences

Exemplars and Baserate Recording Sheet

Print this page from the CD or photocopy this page for your clinical use.

Name/Age:	Date:
Goal: To establish the baserates of the auxiliary *is* in expanded sentences when asked questions while showing a picture or demonstrating an action.	Clinician:

Clinician's Comments:

Scoring: Correct: ✓   Incorrect or no response: X

Auxiliary *is* in Expanded Sentences	Evoked	Modeled
1. The girl is writing a letter.		
2. The woman is walking to her house.		
3. The girl is eating an apple.		
4. The woman is reading a book.		
5. The girl is buying a dress.		
6. The woman is kicking a ball.		
7. The girl is talking on the phone.		
8. The woman is digging dirt.		
9. The boy is sitting on a chair.		
10. The man is cutting the paper.		
11. The boy is opening the box.		
12. The man is cooking dinner.		
13. The boy is building blocks.		
14. The man is sleeping in the bed.		
15. The boy is throwing rocks.		
16. The man is riding a horse.		
17. The bug is moving slowly.		
18. The deer is running fast.		
19. The cat is eating a lot.		
20. The dog is going in circles.		
Percent correct baserate		

Replace or add new exemplars as you see fit for a given child.

After establishing the baserates for the target sentences, initiate treatment. Use the protocols given on the next page.

Auxiliary *is* in Expanded Sentences
Treatment Protocols

Using the following script, teach 8 to 10 sentences with the target auxiliary.

Show a relevant picture or demonstrate a miniature action before you ask the question. Each time, point to the target noun and the action.

Scripts for Modeled Discrete Trial Training		Note
Clinician	"The girl is writing a letter. What is the girl doing? Say, **the girl is writing a letter**."	Vocal emphasis on the target words
Child	"Girl is writing." ["The girl is writing"]	Scored as a wrong response
Clinician	"No, You didn't say the whole sentence. What is the girl doing? Say, **the girl is writing a letter**."	Corrective feedback; vocal emphasis on the target words
Child	"Girl is writing a letter." ["The girl is writing a letter."]	Scored as correct; one or more articles may be included
Clinician	"Very good! You said **girl is writing a letter**!"	Verbal praise

Repeat the trials until the child gives 5 consecutively correct, imitated responses. When the child imitates 5 correct responses in sequence, fade the modeling. Always point to the target object or demonstrate a miniature action before asking a question.

Scripts for Fading the Modeling		Note
Clinician	"The girl is writing a letter. What is the girl doing? Say, the *girl is* . . ."	Partial modeling only
Child	"Writing."	A wrong response
Clinician	"No, you didn't say the whole sentence. *The girl is writing a letter.* What is the girl doing? Say, *the girl is* . . ."	Corrective feedback and partial modeling
Child	"The girl is writing a letter." ["Girl is writing letter."]	A correct response; optional articles may or may not be produced
Clinician	"Very good! You said, *the girl is writing a letter*!"	Verbal praise
Clinician	"What is the girl doing?"	**An Evoked Trial**
Child	"The girl is writing a letter." ["Girl is writing letter."]	Correct answer
Clinician	"Excellent! You said the whole sentence!"	Verbal praise

Auxiliary *is* in Expanded Sentences

Exemplars and Treatment Recording Sheet

Print this page from the CD or photocopy this page for your clinical use.

Name/Age:	Date:
Goal: Production of the auxiliary *is* in expanded sentences with 90% accuracy when asked questions while showing pictures or demonstrating actions.	Clinician:

Clinician's Comments:

Scoring: Correct: ✓   Incorrect or no response: X

Target skills	Discrete Trials														
	1	2	3	4	5	6	7	8	9	10	11	12	13	14	15
1. The girl is writing a letter.															
2. The woman is walking to her house.															
3. The girl is eating an apple.															
4. The woman is reading a book.															
5. The girl is buying a dress.															
6. The woman is kicking a ball.															
7. The girl is talking on the phone.															
8. The woman is digging dirt.															
9. The boy is sitting on a chair.															
10. The man is cutting the paper.															

When the child has met the learning criterion of 10 consecutively correct evoked (nonimitated) responses for each of the 8 to 10 target sentences, conduct a probe to see if the production of the auxiliary has generalized to previously baserated but untrained sentences.

Use the protocol given on the next page (or print it from the CD).

Auxiliary *is* in Expanded Sentences

Probe Protocols and Recording Sheet

Print this page from the CD or photocopy this page for your clinical use.

On the probes, present only the untrained exemplars (UT). When the child fails to meet the 90% correct probe criterion, either teach 2 to 4 new exemplars or give additional training trials on already trained exemplars. If needed, select new exemplars for probes. Probe at least 10 untrained exemplars. Alternate probes and treatment until the probe criterion is met.

Scripts for Probe Trials

Clinician	[Presents an untrained stimulus] "What is the boy doing?"	No modeling or prompts.
Child	"The boy is opening the box." ["Boy is opening box."]	A correct, generalized response
Clinician	Scores the response as correct.	Offers no reinforcement
Clinician	[Presents another untrained stimulus] "What is the man doing?"	The second probe trial
Child	"Man is cooking." ["The man is cooking."]	A wrong probe response
Clinician	Scores the response as incorrect.	Offers no corrective feedback

Name:	**Date:**	**Session #:**
Age:	**Clinician:**	
Disorder: Language	**Target: Auxiliary *is* in Expanded Sentences (Probe)**	
Untrained Stimuli	**Score: + correct; – incorrect or no responses**	
1. The boy is opening the box. (UT)		
2. The man is cooking dinner. (UT)		
3. The boy is building blocks. (UT)		
4. The man is sleeping in the bed. (UT)		
5. The boy is throwing rocks. (UT)		
6. The man is riding a horse. (UT)		
7. The bug is moving slowly. (UT)		
8. The deer is running fast. (UT)		
9. The cat is eating a lot. (UT)		
10. The dog is going in circles. (UT)		
Percent correct probe (Criterion: 90%)		

If the child does not meet the probe criterion, give additional training on already trained sentences and subsequently readminister the probe trials. When the child meets the 90% correct sentence probe criterion for the auxiliary, shift training to other morphologic features or to conversational speech in which the target skills are monitored and reinforced.

Auxiliary *was*
Auxiliary *was* in Basic Sentences
Baserate Protocols

Note that the target sentences include the definite article. The clinician models the phrase with the article, but does not emphasize it or provide contingent consequences (reinforcement or corrective feedback) while teaching the auxiliary. A child may or may not produce the article. Score the responses solely on the basis of presence or absence of the auxiliary. Do not score it incorrect if the child fails to produce the article as it is not the target in this segment of teaching.

Alternatively, the clinician may emphasize the auxiliary as well as the article to teach both at the same time. If this is the clinician's choice, the reinforcement would depend on the production of these two targets.

Scripts for Evoked Baserate Trial		Note
Clinician	[showing the picture of a man or a boy playing with a ball] "He was playing with the ball yesterday. What was he doing yesterday?"	No modeling
Child	"He is playing."	A wrong response
Clinician	Records the response as incorrect.	No corrective feedback
Clinician	[showing the picture of a man or a boy skiing down hill] "He was skiing on the snow last winter. What was he doing on the snow last winter?"	The next trial
Child	"He was skiing."	A correct response; expanded sentence not required
Clinician	Records the response as correct.	No verbal praise

Administer the modeled baserate trials only after completing the evoked trials on all 20 (or more) exemplars.

Scripts for Modeled Baserate Trial		Note
Clinician	[showing the picture of a man or a boy playing with a ball] "He was playing with the ball yesterday. What was he doing yesterday? Say, *he was playing.*"	Modeling
Child	"He playing." ["He was playing."]	A wrong response
Clinician	Records the response as incorrect.	No corrective feedback
Clinician	[showing the picture of a man or a boy skiing down hill] "He was skiing on the snow last winter. What was he doing on the snow last winter? Say, *he was skiing.*"	Modeling
Child	"He was skiing."	A correct response
Clinician	Records the response.	No verbal praise

Baserate at least 20 exemplars as shown on the next page.

Auxiliary *was* in Basic Sentences

Exemplars and Baserate Recording Sheet

Print this page from the CD or photocopy this page for your clinical use.

On modeled trials, model the whole sentence but ignore if the child omits the words given in parentheses.

Name/Age:	Date:
Goal: To establish the baserates of auxiliary *was* in basic sentences when asked questions while showing a picture or demonstrating an action.	Clinician:

Clinician's Comments:

Scoring: Correct: ✓ Incorrect or no response: X

Auxiliary *was* in Basic Sentences	Evoked	Modeled
1. He was playing [with the ball yesterday.]		
2. He was skiing [on the snow last winter.]		
3. She was hopping [on one leg yesterday.]		
4. She was eating [cereal this morning.]		
5. He was cooking [dinner last night.]		
6. He was kicking [a ball last Sunday.]		
7. She was dancing [to music last night.]		
8. She was teaching [painting last year.]		
9. He was fishing [in a lake last summer.]		
10. She was gardening [two days ago.]		
11. He was running [on the grass yesterday.]		
12. He was skipping [on the sidewalk last Saturday.]		
13. He was jumping [rope yesterday.]		
14. She was sailing [in last summer.]		
15. He was sneezing [in class last week.]		
16. He was swimming [in the pool last month.]		
17. She was climbing [a tree yesterday.]		
18. She was riding [a horse last year.]		
19. He was singing [in last year's party.]		
20. She was laughing [at a joke yesterday.]		
Percent correct baserate		

Replace or add exemplars as you see fit to suit an individual child.

Auxiliary *was* in Basic Sentences

Treatment Protocols

At the beginning of each trial, have the child perform a miniature action or place an action picture in front of the child.

Scripts for Modeled Discrete Trial Training		Note
Clinician	[showing the picture of a man or a boy playing with a ball] "He was playing with the ball yesterday. What was he doing yesterday? Say, *he **was** playing*."	Vocal emphasis on the target morpheme
Child	"He playing." ["He is playing."]	A wrong response
Clinician	"No, that is not correct. What was he doing yesterday? Say, *he **was** playing*."	Corrective feedback; vocal emphasis on the target word
Child	"He was playing."	A correct response
Clinician	"Very good! You said *he was playing*!"	Verbal praise

Repeat the trials until the child gives 5 consecutively correct, imitated responses. When the child imitates 5 correct responses in sequence, fade the modeling. Always point to the action picture or perform a miniature action before asking a question.

Scripts for Fading the Modeling		Note
Clinician	"He was playing with the ball yesterday. What was he doing yesterday? Say, *he was . . .*"	Partial modeling only
Child	"He playing." ["Playing.]	A wrong response
Clinician	"No, that is not correct. He was playing with the ball yesterday. What was he doing yesterday? Say, *he was . . .*"	Corrective feedback and partial modeling
Child	"He was playing." ["He was playing yesterday."]	A correct response
Clinician	"Very good! You said *he was playing*!"	Verbal praise
Clinician	"What was he doing yesterday?"	**An Evoked Trial**
Child	"He was playing." ["He was playing yesterday."]	Correct answer

If the wrong responses persist on 4 to 5 evoked trials, reinstate partial or full modeling for a few trials, again fade the modeling, and re-present the evoked trials.

When the child meets the tentative learning criterion of 10 consecutively correct, nonimitated responses for a given exemplar, move on to the next exemplar. With this procedure, teach 8 to 10 exemplars. Use different exemplars as you see fit for a given child. Use the exemplars and the recording sheet given on the next page (or copy it from the CD).

Auxiliary *was* in Basic Sentences

Exemplars and Treatment Recording Sheet

Print this page from the CD or photocopy this page for your clinical use.

Name/Age:	Date:
Goal: Production of the auxiliary *was* in basic sentences with 90% accuracy when asked questions while showing pictures or demonstrating actions.	Clinician:

Clinician's Comments:

Scoring: Correct: ✓   Incorrect or no response: X

Target skills	Discrete Trials														
	1	2	3	4	5	6	7	8	9	10	11	12	13	14	15
1. He was playing [with the ball yesterday.]															
2. He was skiing [on the snow last winter.]															
3. She was hopping [on one leg yesterday.]															
4. She was eating [cereal this morning.]															
5. He was cooking [dinner last night.]															
6. He was kicking [a ball last Sunday.]															
7. She was dancing [to music last night.]															
8. She was teaching [painting last year.]															
9. He was fishing [in a lake last summer.]															
10. She was gardening [two days ago.]															

Teach 8 to 10 exemplars each to a training criterion of 10 consecutively correct, nonimitated responses. Then, baserate expanded sentences and then teach them. Use the protocols that follow.

Auxiliary *was* in Expanded Sentences

Baserate Protocols

Scripts for Evoked Baserate Trial		Note
Clinician	[showing the picture of a boy playing with a ball] "He was playing with the ball yesterday. What was he doing yesterday?"	No modeling
Child	"Playing with ball." ["He was playing ball."]	A wrong response
Clinician	Records the response as incorrect.	No corrective feedback
Clinician	[showing the picture of a man or a boy skiing down hill] "He was skiing on the snow last winter. What was he doing on the snow last winter?"	The next trial
Child	"He was skiing on snow last winter."	A correct response
Clinician	Records the response as correct.	No verbal praise

Administer the modeled baserate trials only after completing the evoked trials on all 20 (or more) exemplars.

Scripts for Modeled Baserate Trial		Note
Clinician	[showing the picture of a man or a boy playing with a ball] "He was playing with the ball yesterday. What was he doing yesterday? Say, *he was playing with the ball yesterday.*"	Modeling
Child	"He playing." ["He is playing."]	A wrong response
Clinician	Records the response as incorrect.	No corrective feedback
Clinician	[showing the picture of a man or a boy skiing down hill] "He was skiing on the snow last winter. What was he doing on the snow last winter? Say, *he was skiing on the snow last winter.*"	Modeling
Child	"He was skiing on snow last winter."	A correct response
Clinician	Records the response.	No verbal praise

Baserate at least 20 exemplars as shown on the next page. Ignore the omission of articles unless previously taught to a training criterion.

Auxiliary *was* in Expanded Sentences

Exemplars and Baserate Recording Sheet

Print this page from the CD or photocopy this page for your clinical use.

Name/Age:	Date:
Goal: To establish the baserates of auxiliary *was* in expanded sentences when asked questions while showing a picture or demonstrating an action.	Clinician:

Clinician's Comments:

Scoring: Correct: ✓ Incorrect or no response: X

Auxiliary *was* in Expanded Sentences	Evoked	Modeled
1. He was playing with the ball yesterday.		
2. He was skiing on the snow last winter.		
3. She was hopping on one leg yesterday.		
4. She was eating cereal this morning.		
5. He was cooking dinner last night.		
6. He was kicking a ball last Sunday.		
7. She was dancing to music last night.		
8. She was teaching painting last year.		
9. He was fishing in a lake last summer.		
10. She was gardening two days ago.		
11. He was running on the grass yesterday.		
12. He was skipping on the sidewalk last Saturday.		
13. He was jumping rope yesterday.		
14. She was sailing last summer.		
15. He was sneezing in class last week.		
16. He was swimming in the pool last month.		
17. She was climbing a tree yesterday.		
18. She was riding a horse last year.		
19. He was singing in last year's party.		
20. She was laughing at a joke yesterday.		
Percent correct baserate		

Replace or add new exemplars as you see fit for a given child.

After establishing the baserates, initiate treatment. Use the protocols given on the next page.

Auxiliary *was* in Expanded Sentences
Treatment Protocols

Teach 8 to10 sentences with the auxiliary was *in sentences using the following script.*

Show a relevant picture before you ask the question. Each time, point to the target noun and the action.

Scripts for Modeled Discrete Trial Training		Note
Clinician	[showing the picture of a man or a boy playing with a ball] "He was playing with the ball yesterday. What was he doing yesterday? Say, *he **was** playing with the ball **yesterday**.*"	Vocal emphasis on the key words
Child	"He was playing ball."	Scored as a wrong response
Clinician	"No, You didn't say the whole sentence. What was he doing? Say, ***he was playing with the ball yesterday.***"	Corrective feedback; vocal emphasis on the target words
Child	"He was playing with the ball yesterday."	Scored as correct; one or more articles may be included
Clinician	"Very good! You said ***he was playing with the ball yesterday**!*"	Verbal raise

Repeat the trials until the child gives 5 consecutively correct, imitated responses. When the child imitates 5 correct responses in sequence, fade the modeling. Always point to the target noun and action before asking a question.

Scripts for Fading the Modeling		Note
Clinician	"He was playing with the ball with yesterday. What was he doing yesterday? Say, *he **was** . . .*"	Partial modeling only
Child	"Playing."	A wrong response
Clinician	"No, you didn't say the whole sentence. *He was playing with the ball yesterday.* What was he doing yesterday? Say, *he was . . .*"	Corrective feedback and partial modeling
Child	"He was playing with the ball yesterday." ["He was playing ball yesterday."]	A correct response; optional articles may or may not be produced
Clinician	"Very good! You said, *he was playing with the ball yesterday*!"	Verbal praise
Clinician	"What was he doing yesterday?"	**An Evoked Trial**
Child	"He was playing with the ball yesterday."	Correct answer
Clinician	"Excellent! You said the whole sentence!"	Verbal praise

Auxiliary *was* in Expanded Sentences

Exemplars and Treatment Recording Sheet

Print this page from the CD or photocopy this page for your clinical use.

Name/Age:	Date:
Goal: Production of the auxiliary *was* in expanded sentences with 90% accuracy when asked questions while showing pictures or demonstrating actions.	Clinician:

Clinician's Comments:

Scoring: Correct: ✓   Incorrect or no response: X

Target skills	Discrete Trials														
	1	2	3	4	5	6	7	8	9	10	11	12	13	14	15
1. He was playing with the ball yesterday.															
2. He was skiing on the snow last winter.															
3. She was hopping on one leg yesterday.															
4. She was eating cereal this morning.															
5. He was cooking dinner last night.															
6. He was kicking a ball last Sunday.															
7. She was dancing to music last night.															
8. She was teaching painting last year.															
9. He was fishing in a lake last summer.															
10. She was gardening two days ago.															

When the child has met the learning criterion of 10 consecutively correct, evoked (nonimitated) responses for each of the 8 to 10 target sentences, conduct a probe to assess generalized production of the auxiliary. Use the protocols given on the next page (or print it from the CD).

Auxiliary *was* in Expanded Sentences

Probe Protocols and Recording Sheet

Print this page from the CD or photocopy this page for your clinical use.

On the probes, present only the untrained exemplars (UT). When the child fails to meet the 90% correct probe criterion, either teach 2 to 4 new exemplars or give additional training trials on already trained exemplars. If needed, select new exemplars for probes. Probe at least 10 untrained exemplars. Alternate probes and treatment until the probe criterion is met.

Scripts for Probe Trials

Clinician	[Presents an untrained stimulus] "What was he doing on the grass yesterday?"	No modeling or prompts
Child	"He was running on the grass yesterday."	A correct, generalized response; the article may be omitted
Clinician	Scores the response as correct.	Offers no reinforcement
Clinician	[Presents another untrained stimulus] "What was he doing on the sidewalk last Saturday?"	The second probe trial
Child	"He was skipping." ["He was skipping yesterday."]	A wrong probe response
Clinician	Scores the response as incorrect.	Offers no corrective feedback

Name:	Date:		Session #:
Age:	Clinician:		
Disorder: Language	Target: Auxiliary *was* in Expanded Sentences (Probe)		
Untrained Stimuli	Score: + correct; – incorrect or no responses		
1. He was running on the grass yesterday.			
2. He was skipping on the sidewalk last Saturday.			
3. He was jumping rope yesterday.			
4. She was sailing last summer.			
5. He was sneezing in class last week.			
6. He was swimming in the pool last month.			
7. She was climbing a tree yesterday.			
8. She was riding a horse last year.			
9. He was singing in last year's party.			
10. She was laughing at a joke yesterday.			
Percent correct probe (Criterion: 90%)			

If the child does not meet the probe criterion, give additional training on already trained sentences and subsequently readminister the probe trials. When the child meets the 90% correct sentence probe criterion for the auxiliary, shift training to other morphologic features or to conversational speech in which the target auxiliary productions are monitored and reinforced.

The Copula

Overview

The English copula is a part of sentences that describe qualities, characteristics, or properties of people and objects. Unlike the auxiliary that helps describe actions and movements, the copula helps describe a state. As noted in the introduction to the auxiliary system, the auxiliary and copula are grammatically different, but behaviorally the same. In other words, auxiliary and copula belong to the same response class. Teaching one is sufficient to have the child produce the other on the basis of generalization. Therefore, if the child has already been taught the auxiliary, the clinician should probe to see if the child produces the copula as well. Most likely the child will. The clinician can offer treatment for copula (or the auxiliary) only if teaching one of them did not result in the generalized production of the other.

General Treatment Strategy

The strategy is the same as that given for the auxiliary. The clinician designs questions to evoke the target sentences with the help of pictures that depict people, animals, and objects with various characteristics described in terms of adjectives.

Copula *is*
Copula *is* in Basic Sentences

Baserate Protocols

Note: *If you already have taught the* **auxiliary is in sentences**, *the child may have mastered the copular form used in similar sentences. Baserates will show whether you need to teach the copula is. If the baserates show 90% or better correct production of the copula, skip training on this feature.*

Important: *While teaching the copular productions, you also teach adjectives. Therefore, to evoke correct responses from the child, use paired contrasting stimuli (e.g., the picture of a big house next to a small house; a funny face drawn next to a sad face). On each trial, point to the target stimulus. A few pretreatment trials in which the pictures are simply contrasted (e.g., "see, this is a big house and this is a small house") may be helpful in directing the child to the target stimulus.*

The basic sentences include the article, but consider its production as optional.

Scripts for Evoked Baserate Trial		Note
Clinician	[showing the picture of a small house and a big house, and pointing to the small one] "Is this house small or big? Start with *the house* . . ."	No modeling, but the correct form is prompted
Child	"House small." ["Small."]	A wrong response
Clinician	Records the response as incorrect.	No corrective feedback
Clinician	[showing the picture of a tall and a short man and pointing to the taller] "Is this man tall or short? Start with, *the man* . . ."	The next trial
Child	"The man is tall." ["Man is tall."]	A correct response; the article may be missing
Clinician	Records the response as correct.	No verbal praise

Administer the modeled baserate trials only after completing the evoked trials on all 20 (or more) exemplars.

Scripts for Modeled Baserate Trial		Note
Clinician	[showing the picture of a small house and a big house, and pointing to the small one] "Is this house small or big? Say, *the house is small.*"	Modeling
Child	"house small." ["Small."]	A wrong response
Clinician	Records the response as incorrect.	No corrective feedback
Clinician	[showing the picture of a tall and a short man, and pointing to the taller] "Is this man tall or short? Say, *the man is tall.*"	Modeling
Child	"The man is tall."	A correct response
Clinician	Records the response.	No verbal praise

Baserate at least 20 exemplars as shown on the next page.

Copula *is* in Basic Sentences

Exemplars and Baserate Recording Sheet

Print this page from the CD or photocopy this page for your clinical use.

Name/Age:	Date:
Goal: To establish the baserates of the copula *is* in basic sentences when asked questions while showing a picture.	Clinician:

Clinician's Comments:

Scoring: Correct: ✓   Incorrect or no response: X

Copula *is* in Basic Sentences	Evoked	Modeled
1. [The] house is small.		
2. [The] man is tall.		
3. [The] turtle is big.		
4. [The] face is funny.		
5. [The] flower is beautiful.		
6. [The] face is happy.		
7. [The] towel is blue.		
8. [The] stove is hot.		
9. [The] ant is small.		
10. [The] boy is thin.		
11. [The] dog is big.		
12. [The] frog is green.		
13. [The] bird is tiny.		
14. [The] boy is sad.		
15. [The] knife is sharp.		
16. [The] candy is sweet.		
17. [The] coat is long.		
18. [The] sink is full.		
19. [The] plant is small.		
20. [The] rabbit is white.		
Percent correct baserate		

Note: *Unless the child has already been taught or has been producing it without teaching, the definite article, shown in brackets above, is optional when teaching the copula.*

After establishing the baserates, initiate treatment. Use the protocols that follow.

Copula *is* in Basic Sentences

Treatment Protocols

At the beginning of each trial, place a single picture that shows contrasting elements or two pictures (e.g., sad and happy faces) in front of the child. Point to the relevant picture as you present the trials.

Scripts for Modeled Discrete Trial Training		Note
Clinician	[showing the picture of a small house and a big house, and pointing to the small one] "Is this house small or big? Say, *the house **is** small.*"	Vocal emphasis on the target morpheme
Child	"Small." ["Small house."]	A wrong response
Clinician	"No, that is not correct. "Is this house small or big? Say, *the house **is** small.*"	Corrective feedback; vocal emphasis on the target word
Child	"House is small." ["The house is small."]	A correct response
Clinician	"Very good! You said *the house **is** small!*"	Verbal praise

Repeat the trials until the child gives 5 consecutively correct, imitated responses. When the child imitates 5 correct responses in sequence, fade the modeling. Always point to the target object before asking a question.

Scripts for Fading the Modeling		Note
Clinician	"The house is small. Is this house small? Say, *the house . . .*"	Partial modeling only
Child	"Small."	A wrong response
Clinician	"No, that is not correct. The house is small. Is the house small? Say, *the house . . .*"	Corrective feedback and partial modeling
Child	"The house is small." ["House is small."]	A correct response
Clinician	"Very good! You said *the house **is** small!*"	Verbal praise
Clinician	"Is the house small?"	**An Evoked Trial**
Child	"The house is small." ["House is small."]	Correct answer; if the child were to say "yes," prompt to "start with *the house.*"

If the wrong responses persist on 4 to 5 evoked trials, reinstate partial or full modeling for a few trials, again fade the modeling, and re-present the evoked trials.

When the child meets the tentative learning criterion of 10 consecutively correct, nonimitated responses for a given exemplar, move on to the next exemplar. With this procedure, teach 8 to 10 exemplars. Use different exemplars as you see fit for a given child. Use the exemplars and the recording sheet given on the next page (or print it from the CD).

Copula *is* in Basic Sentences

Exemplars and Treatment Recording Sheet

Print this page from the CD or photocopy this page for your clinical use.

Name/Age:	Date:
Goal: Production of the copula *is* in basic sentences with 90% accuracy when asked questions while showing pictures.	Clinician:

Clinician's Comments:

Scoring: Correct: ✓   Incorrect or no response: X

Target skills	Discrete Trials														
	1	2	3	4	5	6	7	8	9	10	11	12	13	14	15
1. [The] house is small.															
2. [The] man is tall.															
3. [The] turtle is big.															
4. [The] face is funny.															
5. [The] flower is beautiful.															
6. [The] face is happy.															
7. [The] towel is blue.															
8. [The] stove is hot.															
9. [The] ant is small.															
10. [The] boy is thin.															

Teach 8 to 10 basic sentence exemplars each to a training criterion of 10 consecutively correct, non-imitated responses. Then, shift training to the expanded sentence level. Before teaching the copula in expanded sentences, baserate their productions. Use the protocols that follow.

Copula *is* in Expanded Sentences
Baserate Protocols

On each trial, use paired pictures with contrasting elements.

Scripts for Evoked Baserate Trial		Note
Clinician	[showing the picture of a small house and a big house, and pointing to the small one] "Is this house big or small? Start with, *this house . . .*"	No modeling, but prompting the response
Child	"House is small." ["House small."]	A wrong response
Clinician	Records the response as incorrect.	No corrective feedback
Clinician	[showing the picture of a tall man and a short man, and pointing to the tall man] "Is this man tall or short? Start with, *this man . . .*"	The next trial
Child	"This man is tall."	A correct response
Clinician	Records the response as correct.	No verbal praise

Administer the modeled baserate trials only after completing the evoked trials on all 20 (or more) exemplars.

Scripts for Modeled Baserate Trial		Note
Clinician	[showing the picture of a small house and a big house, and pointing to the small one] "Is this house big or small? Say, *this house **is** small.*"	Modeling
Child	"House is small."	A wrong response
Clinician	Records the response as incorrect.	No corrective feedback
Clinician	[showing the picture of a tall man and a short man, and pointing to the tall man] "Is this man short or tall? Say, *this man is tall.*"	Modeling
Child	"This man is tall."	A correct response
Clinician	Records the response.	No verbal praise

Baserate at least 20 exemplars as shown on the next page.

Copula *is* in Expanded Sentences

Exemplars and Baserate Recording Sheet

Print this page from the CD or photocopy this page for your clinical use.

Name/Age:	Date:
Goal: To establish the baserates of copula *is* in expanded sentences when asked questions while showing a picture.	Clinician:

Clinician's Comments:

Scoring: Correct: ✓   Incorrect or no response: X

Copula *is* in Expanded Sentences	Evoked	Modeled
1. This house is small.		
2. This man is tall.		
3. This turtle is big.		
4. This face is funny.		
5. This flower is beautiful.		
6. This face is happy.		
7. This towel is blue.		
8. This stove is hot.		
9. This ant is small.		
10. This boy is thin.		
11. This dog is big.		
12. This frog is green.		
13. This bird is tiny.		
14. This boy is sad.		
15. This knife is sharp.		
16. This candy is sweet.		
17. This coat is long.		
18. This sink is full.		
19. This plant is small.		
20. This rabbit is white.		
Percent correct baserate		

Replace or add new exemplars as you see fit for a given child.

After establishing the baserates for the target sentences, initiate treatment. Use the protocols given on the next page.

Copula *is* in Expanded Sentences

Treatment Protocols

Teach 8 to 10 sentences with the copula is in sentences using the following script.

Point to the relevant pictures before you ask the question.

Scripts for Modeled Discrete Trial Training		Note
Clinician	[showing the picture of a small house and a big house, and pointing to the small one] "Is this house big or small? Say, **this** house **is** small."	Vocal emphasis on the target words
Child	"House is small." ["small house."]	Scored as a wrong response
Clinician	"No, You didn't say the whole sentence. Is this house big or small? Say, **this** house **is** small."	Corrective feedback; vocal emphasis on the target words
Child	"This house is small."	Scored as correct
Clinician	"Very good! You said **this** house **is** small!"	Verbal praise

Repeat the trials until the child gives 5 consecutively correct, imitated responses. When the child imitates 5 correct responses in sequence, fade the modeling. Always point to the target object before asking a question.

Scripts for Fading the Modeling		Note
Clinician	"Is this house big or small? Say, *this house . . . "*	Partial modeling only
Child	"Small."	A wrong response
Clinician	"No, you didn't say the whole sentence. Is this house big or small? Say, *this house . . . "*	Corrective feedback and partial modeling
Child	"This house is small."	A correct response
Clinician	"Very good! You said, *this house is small!"*	Verbal praise
Clinician	"Is this house big or small?"	**An Evoked Trial**
Child	"This house is small."	Correct answer
Clinician	"Excellent! You said the whole sentence!"	Verbal praise

Copula *is* in Expanded Sentences

Exemplars and Treatment Recording Sheet

Print this page from the CD or photocopy this page for your clinical use.

Name/Age:	Date:
Goal: Production of the copula *is* in expanded sentences with 90% accuracy when asked questions while showing pictures.	Clinician:

Clinician's Comments:

Scoring: Correct: ✓   Incorrect or no response: X

Target skills	Discrete Trials														
	1	2	3	4	5	6	7	8	9	10	11	12	13	14	15
1. This house is small.															
2. This man is tall.															
3. This turtle is big.															
4. This face is funny.															
5. This flower is beautiful.															
6. This face is happy.															
7. This towel is blue.															
8. This stove is hot.															
9. This ant is small.															
10. This boy is thin.															

When the child has met the learning criterion of 10 consecutively correct, evoked (nonimitated) responses for each of the 8 to 10 target sentences, conduct a probe to see if the production of the copula has generalized to previously baserated but untrained sentences.

Use the protocols given on the next page (or print it from the CD).

Copula *is* in Expanded Sentences

Probe Protocols and Recording Sheet

Print this page from the CD or photocopy this page for your clinical use.

On the probes, present only the untrained exemplars (UT). When the child fails to meet the 90% correct probe criterion, either teach 2 to 4 new exemplars or give additional training trials on already trained exemplars. If needed, select new exemplars for probes. Probe at least 10 untrained exemplars. Alternate probes and treatment until the probe criterion is met.

Scripts for Probe Trials

Clinician	[Presents an untrained stimulus pair] "Is this dog small or big?"	No modeling or prompts
Child	"This dog is big.	A correct, generalized response
Clinician	Scores the response as correct.	Offers no reinforcement
Clinician	[Presents another untrained stimulus] "Is this frog black or green?"	The second probe trial
Child	"Frog is green."	A wrong probe response
Clinician	Scores the response as incorrect.	Offers no corrective feedback

Name:	Date:	Session #:
Age:	**Clinician:**	
Disorder: Language	**Target: Copula *is* in Expanded Sentences (Probe)**	
Untrained Stimuli	**Score: + correct; – incorrect or no responses**	
1. This dog is big. (UT)		
2. This frog is green. (UT)		
3. This bird is tiny. (UT)		
4. This boy is sad. (UT)		
5. This knife is sharp. (UT)		
6. This candy is sweet. (UT)		
7. This coat is long. (UT)		
8. This sink is full. (UT)		
9. This plant is small. (UT)		
10. This rabbit is white. (UT)		
Percent correct probe (Criterion: 90%)		

If the child does not meet the probe criterion, give additional training on already trained sentences and subsequently readminister the probe trials. When the child meets the 90% correct sentence probe criterion for the copula, shift training to other morphologic features or to conversational speech in which the target skills are monitored and reinforced.

Copula *was*
Copula *was* in Basic Sentences
Baserate Protocols

Note: *If you already have taught the auxiliary was in sentences, the child may have mastered the copular form used in similar sentences. If the baserates show 90% or better correct production of the copula* was, *skip training on this feature.*

Important: *While teaching the copular productions, you also teach adjectives. Therefore, to evoke correct responses from the child, use paired contrasting stimuli (e.g., the picture of a happy face and a sad face). On each trial, point to the target stimulus. A few pretreatment trials on which the pictures are simply contrasted (e.g., "see, this was a new car and now it is an old car") may be helpful in directing the children to the target stimulus.*

Scripts for Evoked Baserate Trial		Note
Clinician	[showing the picture of a man's mad face and a smiling face, and pointing to the appropriate face] "He is happy now, but he was mad before. Was he happy or mad? Start with *he . . .* "	No modeling
Child	"He mad." ["Mad."]	A wrong response
Clinician	Records the response as incorrect.	No corrective feedback
Clinician	[showing the picture of a young and an old face of the same man, and pointing to the appropriate face] "He is old now, but he was young before. Was he old or young? Start with *he . . .* "	The next trial
Child	"He was young."	A correct response
Clinician	Records the response as correct.	No verbal praise

Administer the modeled baserate trials only after completing the evoked trials on all 20 (or more) exemplars.

Scripts for Modeled Baserate Trial		Note
Clinician	[showing the picture and pointing to the appropriate face] "He is happy now, but he was mad before. Was he happy or mad? Say, *he was mad.*"	Modeling
Child	"He mad." ["Mad."]	A wrong response
Clinician	Records the response as incorrect.	No corrective feedback
Clinician	[showing the picture of a young and an old face of the same man, and pointing to the appropriate face] "He is old now, but he was young before. Was he old or young? Say, *he was old.*"	Modeling
Child	"He was old."	A correct response
Clinician	Records the response.	No verbal praise

Baserate at least 20 exemplars as shown on the next page.

Copula *was* in Basic Sentences

Exemplars and Baserate Recording Sheet

Print this page from the CD or photocopy this page for your clinical use.

Replace or add exemplars as you see fit to suit an individual child.

Name/Age:	Date:
Goal: To establish the baserates of the copula *was* in basic sentences when asked questions while showing pictures.	Clinician:

Clinician's Comments:

Scoring: Correct: ✓   Incorrect or no response: X

Copula *was* in Basic Sentences	Evoked	Modeled
1. He was mad.		
2. He was young.		
3. He was clean.		
4. He was happy.		
5. She was neat.		
6. She was hungry.		
7. She was sad.		
8. She was small.		
9. This was smooth.		
10. This was soft.		
11. This was yellow.		
12. This was round.		
13. This was full.		
14. This was long.		
15. This was a puppy.		
16. This was green.		
17. It was new.		
18. It was wet.		
19. It was white.		
20. It was friendly.		
Percent correct baserate		

After establishing the baserates, initiate treatment. Use the protocols that follow.

Copula *was* in Basic Sentences

Treatment Protocols

At the beginning of each trial, place a single picture that shows contrasting elements or two pictures (e.g., a young and an old face of the same person). Point to the relevant picture as you present the trials.

Scripts for Modeled Discrete Trial Training		Note
Clinician	[showing the picture and pointing to the appropriate face] "He is happy now, but he was mad before. Was he happy or mad? Say, *he **was** mad.*"	Vocal emphasis on the target morpheme
Child	"He mad." ["Mad."]	A wrong response
Clinician	"No, that is not correct. "was he happy or mad? Say, *he **was** mad.*"	Corrective feedback; vocal emphasis on the target word
Child	"He was mad."	A correct response
Clinician	"Very good! You said *he **was** mad!*"	Verbal praise

Repeat the trials until the child gives 5 consecutively correct, imitated responses. When the child imitates 5 correct responses in sequence, fade the modeling. Always point to the target object before asking a question.

Scripts for Fading the Modeling		Note
Clinician	"He is happy now, but he was mad before. Was he happy or mad? Say, *he . . .* "	Partial modeling only
Child	"Mad." ["Happy."]	A wrong response
Clinician	"No, that is not correct. He was mad. Was he happy or mad? Say, *he . . .*"	Corrective feedback and partial modeling
Child	"He was mad."	A correct response
Clinician	"Very good! You said *he was mad!*"	Verbal praise
Clinician	"Was he happy or mad?"	**An Evoked Trial**
Child	"He was mad."	Correct answer; if the child were to say, "yes," prompt to "start with *he was.*"

If the wrong responses persist on 4 to 5 evoked trials, reinstate partial or full modeling for a few trials, again fade the modeling, and re-present the evoked trials.

When the child meets the tentative learning criterion of 10 consecutively correct, nonimitated responses for a given exemplar, move on to the next exemplar. With this procedure, teach 8 to 10 exemplars. Use different exemplars as you see fit for a given child. Use the exemplars and the recording sheet given on the next page (or copy it from the CD).

Copula *was* in Basic Sentences

Exemplars and Treatment Recording Sheet

Print this page from the CD or photocopy this page for your clinical use.

Name/Age:	Date:
Goal: Production of the copula *was* in basic sentences with 90% accuracy when asked questions while showing pictures.	Clinician:

Clinician's Comments:

Scoring: Correct: ✓   Incorrect or no response: X

Target skills	Discrete Trials														
	1	2	3	4	5	6	7	8	9	10	11	12	13	14	15
1. He was mad.															
2. He was young.															
3. He was clean.															
4. He was happy.															
5. She was neat.															
6. She was hungry.															
7. She was sad.															
8. She was small.															
9. This was smooth.															
10. This was soft.															

Teach 8 to 10 basic sentence exemplars each to a training criterion of 10 consecutively correct, non-imitated responses. Then, shift training to the expanded sentence level. Before teaching the copula in expanded sentences, baserate their productions. Use the protocols that follow.

Copula *was* in Expanded Sentences

Baserating Protocols

On each trial, use paired pictures with contrasting elements.

Scripts for Evoked Baserate Trial		Note
Clinician	[showing the picture of a man's mad face and a smiling face, and pointing to the appropriate face] "He is happy now, but he was mad before. Was he happy or mad before? Start with *he*."	No modeling
Child	"He was mad." ["He mad."]	A wrong response
Clinician	Records the response as incorrect.	No corrective feedback
Clinician	[showing the picture of a young and an old face of the same man, and pointing to the appropriate face] "He is old now, but he was young before. Was he old or young? Start with *he*."	The next trial
Child	"He was young before."	A correct response
Clinician	Records the response as correct.	No verbal praise

Administer the modeled baserate trials only after completing the evoked trials on all 20 (or more) exemplars.

Scripts for Modeled Baserate Trial		Note
Clinician	[pointing to the appropriate pictures] "He is happy now, but he was mad before. Was he happy or mad before? Say, *he was mad before*."	Modeling
Child	"He was mad."	A wrong response
Clinician	Records the response as incorrect.	No corrective feedback
Clinician	[Pointing to the appropriate pictures] "He is old now, but he was young before. Was he old or young before? Say, *he was young before*."	Modeling
Child	"He was young before."	A correct response
Clinician	Records the response.	No verbal praise

Baserate at least 20 exemplars as shown on the next page.

Copula *was* in Expanded Sentences

Exemplars and Baserate Recording Sheet

Print this page from the CD or photocopy this page for your clinical use.

Name/Age:	Date:
Goal: To establish the baserates of the copula *was* in expanded sentences when asked questions while showing pictures.	Clinician:

Clinician's Comments:

Scoring: Correct: ✓   Incorrect or no response: X

Copula *was* in Expanded Sentences	Evoked	Modeled
1. He was mad before.		
2. He was young before.		
3. He was clean yesterday.		
4. He was happy before.		
5. She was a neat woman.		
6. She was a hungry woman.		
7. She was sad before.		
8. She was small before.		
9. This was a thin book.		
10. This was a soft doll.		
11. This was a yellow flower.		
12. This was a round pizza.		
13. This was a full cup.		
14. This was a long bat.		
15. This was a white puppy.		
16. This was a green tree.		
17. It was a new car.		
18. It was a wet bird.		
19. It was a white shirt.		
20. It was a friendly lion.		
Percent correct baserate		

Replace or add new exemplars as you see fit for a given child.

After establishing the baserates for the target sentences, initiate treatment. Use the protocols given on the next page.

Copula *was* in Expanded Sentences

Treatment Protocols

Teach 8 to 10 sentences with the copula was *using the following script.*

Point to the relevant pictures before you ask the question.

Scripts for Modeled Discrete Trial Training		Note
Clinician	[pointing to the appropriate pictures] "He is happy now, but he was mad before. Was he happy or mad before? Say, **he was** *mad before*."	Vocal emphasis on the target words
Child	"He was mad." ["Mad before."]	Scored as a wrong response
Clinician	"No, You didn't say the whole sentence. Was he happy or mad before? Say, **he was** *mad before*."	Corrective feedback; vocal emphasis on the target words
Child	"He was mad before."	Scored as correct
Clinician	"Very good! You said **he was** *mad before*!"	Verbal praise

Repeat the trials until the child gives 5 consecutively correct, imitated responses. When the child imitates 5 correct responses in sequence, fade the modeling. Always point to the target object before asking a question.

Scripts for Fading the Modeling		Note
Clinician	[pointing to the appropriate pictures] "Was he happy or mad? Say, *he . . .* "	Partial modeling only
Child	"Was mad." ("Mad")	A wrong response
Clinician	"No, you didn't say the whole sentence. Was he happy or mad? Say, *he . . .* "	Corrective feedback and partial modeling
Child	"He was mad before."	A correct response
Clinician	"Very good! You said, *he was mad before*!"	Verbal praise
Clinician	"Was he happy or mad?"	**An Evoked Trial**
Child	"He was mad before."	Correct answer
Clinician	"Excellent! You said the whole sentence!"	Verbal praise

Copula *was* in Expanded Sentences

Exemplars and Treatment Recording Sheet

Print this page from the CD or photocopy this page for your clinical use.

Name/Age:	Date:
Goal: Production of the copula *was* in expanded sentences with 90% accuracy when asked questions while showing pictures.	Clinician:

Clinician's Comments:

Scoring: Correct: ✓   Incorrect or no response: X

Target skills	Discrete Trials														
	1	2	3	4	5	6	7	8	9	10	11	12	13	14	15
1. He was mad before.															
2. He was young before.															
3. He was clean yesterday.															
4. He was happy before.															
5. She was a neat woman.															
6. She was a hungry woman.															
7. She was sad before.															
8. She was small before.															
9. This was a thin book.															
10. This was a soft doll.															

When the child has met the learning criterion of 10 consecutively correct, evoked (nonimitated) responses for each of the 8 to 10 target sentences, conduct a probe to see if the production of the copula has generalized to previously baserated but untrained sentences.

Use the protocol given on the next page (or print it from the CD).

Copula *was* in Expanded Sentences

Probe Protocols and Recording Sheet

Print this page from the CD or photocopy this page for your clinical use.

On the probes, present the untrained exemplars (UT). When the child fails to meet the 90% correct probe criterion, either teach 2 to 4 new exemplars or give additional training trials on already trained exemplars. If needed, select new exemplars for probes. Probe at least 10 untrained exemplars. Alternate probes and treatment until the probe criterion is met.

Scripts for Probe Trials

Clinician	[Presents an untrained stimulus pair] "Was this a yellow flower? Start with *this*"	No modeling, only a prompt
Child	"This was a yellow flower."	A correct, generalized response
Clinician	Scores the response as correct.	Offers no reinforcement
Clinician	[Presents another untrained stimulus pair] "Was this a round pizza?"	The second probe trial
Child	"Round pizza." ["Yes."]	A wrong probe response
Clinician	Scores the response as incorrect.	Offers no corrective feedback

Name:	Date:	Session #:	
Age:	**Clinician:**		
Disorder: Language	**Target: Copula *was* in Expanded Sentences (Probe)**		
Untrained Stimuli	**Score: + correct; – incorrect or no responses**		
1. This was a yellow flower. (UT)	
2. This was a round pizza. (UT)	
3. This was a full cup. (UT)	
4. This was a long bat. (UT)	
5. This was a white puppy. (UT)	
6. This was a green tree. (UT)	
7. It was a new car. (UT)	
8. It was a wet bird. (UT)	
9. It was a white shirt. (UT)	
10. It was a friendly lion. (UT)	
Percent correct probe (Criterion: 90%)	

If the child does not meet the probe criterion, give additional training on already trained sentences and subsequently readminister the probe trials. When the child meets the 90% correct sentence probe criterion for the copula, shift training to other morphologic features or to conversational speech in which the target skills are monitored and reinforced.

Past Tenses

Overview

Tense-marking morphemes are important targets for children with language disorders. Missing tense markers is a characteristic of child language disorders. Understanding temporal relationships between events is essential to correctly and spontaneously produce the tense-marking morphemes. In Brown's (1973) classic study, children mastered irregular past words before they mastered the allomorphic variations of the regular past tense marker.

Similar to the plural morpheme, the past tense marker is a complex morphologic skill. Structurally, it includes the regular and the irregular varieties. Functionally, it is more than the two structural categories. The past tense maker is a collection of functional response classes. Each irregular past tense word is a response class unto itself; each word has to be taught separately. Teaching a few irregular past words (e.g., *ate* and *went*) will not result in generalized production of other words (e.g., *broke* and *came*). The regular past, though a single structural category, breaks down into multiple response classes, each to be taught separately. For example, the clinician will have to teach the past tense *d* inflection (e.g., *cried*, *pulled*), *t* inflection (e.g., *baked*, *dropped*), and *ed* inflection (e.g., *folded*, *painted*) separately.

General Training Strategy

Pictures serve well in teaching the production of tense-marking morphemes. For certain words, the clinician may add words that signal temporal relations to her model (e.g., "*Yesterday, the bird flew; Last year, he painted the house*"). The clinician can stop teaching when a set of functional words has been taught.

In most cases, teaching may begin at the phrase or even at the word level, depending on the child's response rate. If needed, the clinician can give a few modeled training trials at the word level (e.g., "Say, *ate*"; "Say, *went*") to familiarize the child with the task and to orient the child to the target. The clinician can then swiftly move on to the phrase or sentence level.

Probes for irregular past morphemes are similar to those of irregular plural morphemes and are different from probes for most other morphemes. See probe protocols for details.

Irregular Past Morphemes
Irregular Past Morphemes in Basic Sentences
Baserate Protocols

Administer the evoked trials first followed by modeled trials. Do not provide feedback on any trials; just record the responses on the recording sheet provided on the next page or printed from the CD.

Scripts for Evoked Baserate Trial		Note
Clinician	[showing the picture of a boy eating pizza] "This boy is eating pizza now, but he also ate a pizza yesterday. What did the boy do yesterday?"	No modeling
Child	"Boy eat." ["Boy eat pizza."]	A wrong response
Clinician	Records the response as incorrect.	No corrective feedback
Clinician	[showing the picture of a broken toy] "This girl broke this toy. What did the girl do?"	The next trial
Child	"Girl broke toy." ["Broke toy"]	A correct response
Clinician	Records the response as correct.	No verbal praise

Administer the modeled baserate trials only after completing the evoked trials on all 20 (or more) exemplars.

Scripts for Modeled Baserate Trial		Note
Clinician	[showing the picture of a boy eating pizza] "This boy is eating pizza now, but he also ate a pizza yesterday. What did the boy do yesterday? Say, *the boy ate pizza.*"	Modeling
Child	"Boy eat." ["Boy eat pizza."]	A wrong response
Clinician	Records the response as incorrect.	No corrective feedback
Clinician	[showing the picture of a broken toy] "This girl broke this toy. What did the girl do? Say, *the girl broke the toy.*"	Modeling
Child	"Girl broke toy."	A correct response; one or more articles may be missing
Clinician	Records the response.	No verbal praise

Baserate at least 20 exemplars as shown on the next page.

Irregular Past Morphemes in Basic Sentences

Exemplars and Baserate Recording Sheet

Print this page from the CD or photocopy this page for your clinical use.

Replace or add exemplars as you see fit to suit an individual child. Consider the production of the article in parentheses as optional.

Name/Age:		Date:
Goal: To establish the baserates of irregular past morphemes in basic sentences when asked questions while showing a picture.		Clinician:

Clinician's Comments:

Scoring: Correct: ✓   Incorrect or no response: X

Irregular Past in Basic Sentences	Evoked	Modeled
1. [The] boy ate pizza.		
2. [The] girl broke the toy.		
3. [The] baby fell down.		
4. [The] man caught the ball.		
5. She came home.		
6. [The] doggie swam in pool.		
7. [The] girl found the ball.		
8. [The] boy built a tower.		
9. [The] man slept on the sofa.		
10. [The] boy hid the car.		
11. [The] bird flew away.		
12. She rode the bus.		
13. [The] boy brought a kitty.		
14. [The] teacher gave gift.		
15. He sat on the chair.		
16. Mommy fed the baby.		
17. He threw the ball.		
18. He swept the floor.		
19. Yesterday he went to the store.		
20. Yesterday the baby drank milk.		
Percent correct baserate		

After establishing the baserates, initiate treatment. Use the protocols that follow.

Irregular Past Morphemes in Basic Sentences
Treatment Protocols

Important: *Give a few modeled trials at the phrase level if the child has difficulty imitating sentences that contain the irregular past tense words. If needed, give a detailed background information. For example, give instructions like the following:*

> *"We will work on a few words that help you talk about what happened sometime ago, like yesterday, day before yesterday, or even last year. See, in this picture, the boy is eating pizza. But he did the same yesterday. He ate pizza yesterday. What did he do yesterday? Say, he ate. [he ate pizza]."*

Such detailed background information may be repeated on a few initial trials and periodically given as found necessary. It may not be needed on every trial, however.

Scripts for Modeled Discrete Trial Training		Note
Clinician	[showing the picture of a boy eating pizza] "This boy is eating pizza now, but he also ate pizza yesterday. What did the boy do yesterday? Say, *the boy ate pizza.*"	Vocal emphasis on the target morpheme
Child	"Boy eat." ["Boy eat pizza."]	A wrong response
Clinician	"No, that is not correct. The boy ate pizza yesterday. Say, *the boy **ate** pizza.*"	Corrective feedback; vocal emphasis on the target word
Child	"Boy ate pizza."	A correct response
Clinician	"Very good! You said *boy **ate** pizza!*"	Verbal praise

Repeat the trials until the child gives 5 consecutively correct, imitated responses. When the child imitates 5 correct responses in sequence, fade the modeling. Always point to the target object before asking a question.

Scripts for Fading the Modeling		Note
Clinician	"The boy is eating now, but the boy also ate yesterday. What did the boy do yesterday? Say, *the boy . . .*"	Partial modeling only
Child	"Eating" ["Eating pizza."]	A wrong response
Clinician	"No, that is not correct. The boy ate yesterday. What did the boy do yesterday? Say, *the boy . . .*"	Corrective feedback and partial modeling
Child	"The boy ate pizza."	A correct response
Clinician	"Very good! You said *the boy ate pizza!*"	Verbal praise
Clinician	"What did the boy do yesterday?"	**An Evoked Trial**
Child	"The boy ate pizza." ["The boy ate pizza yesterday."]	Correct answer; the article may be missing

If the wrong responses persist on 4 to 5 evoked trials, reinstate partial or full modeling for a few trials, again fade the modeling, and re-present the evoked trials.

When the child meets the tentative learning criterion of 10 consecutively correct, nonimitated responses for a given exemplar, move on to the next exemplar. With this procedure, teach 8 to 10 exemplars. Use different exemplars as you see fit for a given child. Use the exemplars and the recording sheet given on the next page (or print it from the CD).

Irregular Past Morphemes in Basic Sentences

Exemplars and Treatment Recording Sheet

Print this page from the CD or photocopy this page for your clinical use.

Teach a set of functional exemplars using the previous scripts. To teach additional irregular plural words, print this page from the CD and type in new exemplars (of the kind given on the Baserate Recording Sheet).

Name/Age:	Date:
Goal: Production of the irregular past morphemes in basic sentences with 90% accuracy when asked questions while showing pictures.	Clinician:

Clinician's Comments:

Scoring: Correct: ✓   Incorrect or no response: X

Target skills	Discrete Trials														
	1	2	3	4	5	6	7	8	9	10	11	12	13	14	15
1. [The] boy ate pizza.															
2. [The] girl broke the toy.															
3. [The] baby fell down.															
4. [The] man caught the ball.															
5. She came home.															
6. [The] doggie swam in pool.															
7. [The] girl found the ball.															
8. [The] boy built a tower.															
9. [The] man slept on the sofa.															
10. [The] boy hid the car.															

Teach a set of basic functional sentence exemplars each to a training criterion of 10 consecutively correct nonimitated responses. Then, shift training to the expanded sentence level. Before teaching the irregular past words in expanded sentences, baserate their productions. Use the protocols that follow.

Irregular Past Morphemes in Expanded Sentences

Baserate Protocols

On each trial, use paired pictures with contrasting elements.

Scripts for Evoked Baserate Trial		Note
Clinician	[showing the picture of a boy eating pizza] "This boy is eating pizza now, but he also ate pizza yesterday. What did the boy do yesterday?"	No modeling
Child	"The boy ate." ["The boy ate pizza"]	A wrong response
Clinician	Records the response as incorrect.	No corrective feedback
Clinician	[showing the picture of a broken toy] "This girl broke this toy earlier. What did the girl do earlier?"	The next trial
Child	"Girl broke toy earlier."	A correct response; articles may be produced or not
Clinician	Records the response as correct.	No verbal praise

Administer the modeled baserate trials only after completing the evoked trials on all 20 (or more) exemplars.

Scripts for Modeled Baserate Trial		Note
Clinician	[showing the picture of a boy eating pizza] "This boy is eating pizza now, but he also ate a pizza yesterday. What did the boy do yesterday? Say, *the boy ate pizza yesterday.*"	Modeling
Child	"Boy ate." ["Boy eat pizza."]	A wrong response
Clinician	Records the response as incorrect.	No corrective feedback
Clinician	[showing the picture of a broken toy] "This girl broke this toy earlier. What did the girl do earlier? Say, *the girl broke the toy earlier.*"	Modeling
Child	"Girl broke toy earlier."	A correct response; articles may be missing
Clinician	Records the response.	No verbal praise

Baserate at least 20 exemplars as shown on the next page.

Irregular Past Morphemes in Expanded Sentences
Exemplars and Baserate Recording Sheet

Print this page from the CD or photocopy this page for your clinical use.

Name/Age:	Date:
Goal: To establish the baserates of irregular past morphemes in expanded sentences when asked questions while showing a picture.	Clinician:

Clinician's Comments:

Scoring: Correct: ✓   Incorrect or no response: X

Irregular Past Morphemes in Expanded Sentences	Evoked	Modeled
1. The boy ate pizza yesterday.		
2. The girl broke the toy earlier.		
3. The baby fell down last night.		
4. The man caught the ball fast.		
5. She came home from work.		
6. The doggie swam in the cold pool.		
7. The girl found the ball in the box.		
8. The boy built a tall tower.		
9. Man slept on the sofa last night.		
10. The boy hid the car under the table.		
11. The bird flew away to its nest.		
12. She rode the bus to the school.		
13. The boy brought a kitty home.		
14. The teacher gave gift to the girl.		
15. He sat on the big chair.		
16. Mommy fed the hungry baby.		
17. He threw the ball to the boy.		
18. He swept the floor clean.		
19. He went to the store to get cookies.		
20. The baby drank milk from the bottle.		
Percent correct baserate		

Replace or add new exemplars as you see fit for a given child.

After establishing the baserates for the target sentences, initiate treatment. Use the protocols given on the next page.

Irregular Past Morphemes in Expanded Sentences

Treatment Protocols

Teach a set of functional sentences with the irregular plural words using the following script. Point to the relevant action pictures before you ask the question.

Scripts for Modeled Discrete Trial Training		Note
Clinician	[showing the picture of a boy eating pizza] "This boy is eating pizza now, but he also ate pizza yesterday. What did the boy do yesterday? Say, *the boy **ate** pizza yesterday.*"	Vocal emphasis on the target word
Child	"Ate pizza." ["Ate pizza yesterday."]	Scored as a wrong response
Clinician	"No, you didn't say the whole sentence. What did the boy do yesterday? Say, the boy ***ate*** *pizza yesterday.*"	Corrective feedback; vocal emphasis on the target word
Child	"The boy ate pizza yesterday."	Scored as correct; the article may be missing
Clinician	"Very good! You said the boy ***ate*** *pizza yesterday*!"	Verbal praise

Repeat the trials until the child gives 5 consecutively correct, imitated responses. When the child imitates 5 correct responses in sequence, fade the modeling. Always point to the target action before asking a question.

Scripts for Fading the Modeling		Note
Clinician	[pointing to the appropriate pictures] "What did the boy do yesterday? Say, *The boy . . .*"	Partial modeling only
Child	"Ate pizza." ("Ate pizza yesterday.")	A wrong response
Clinician	"No, you didn't say the whole sentence. What did the boy do yesterday? Say, *the boy . . .*"	Corrective feedback and partial modeling
Child	"The boy ate pizza yesterday."	A correct response
Clinician	"Very good! You said, *the boy ate pizza yesterday*!"	Verbal praise
Clinician	"What did the boy do yesterday?"	**An Evoked Trial**
Child	"The boy ate pizza yesterday."	Correct answer
Clinician	"Excellent! You said the whole sentence!"	Verbal praise

Irregular Past Morphemes in Expanded Sentences
Exemplars and Treatment Recording Sheet

Print this page from the CD or photocopy this page for your clinical use.

Name/Age:	Date:
Goal: Production of the irregular past morphemes in expanded sentences with 90% accuracy when asked questions while showing action pictures.	Clinician:

Clinician's Comments:

Scoring: Correct: ✓   Incorrect or no response: X

Target skills	Discrete Trials														
	1	2	3	4	5	6	7	8	9	10	11	12	13	14	15
1. [The] boy ate pizza yesterday.															
2. [The] girl broke the toy earlier.															
3. [The] baby fell down last night.															
4. [The] man caught the ball fast.															
5. She came home from work.															
6. [The] doggie swam in the cold pool.															
7. [The] girl found the ball in the box.															
8. [The] boy built a tall tower.															
9. [The] man slept on the sofa last night.															
10. [The] boy hid the car under the table.															

When the child has met the learning criterion of 10 consecutively correct, evoked (nonimitated) responses for each of the 10 target sentences, conduct a probe to see if the production of each word generalizes to different kinds of pictures—not used in training—but designed to evoke the same irregular plural word.

Use the protocols and the recording sheet given on the next page (or print it from the CD).

Irregular Past Morphemes in Expanded Sentences

Probe Protocols and Recording Sheet

Print this page from the CD or photocopy this page for your clinical use.

Important: *The nature of generalized productions is unique for the irregular plural words. There is no generalization within this structural category; that is, learning one irregular plural word has no effect on other irregular plural words. The clinician needs to teach as many irregular past morphemes as is considered essential for a given child's academic and social communication. On the probes, new (untrained) stimuli (UT) are presented to evoke the same trained response. Therefore, the probe recording sheet includes the same trained responses. To evoke the same trained response (e.g., ate), the clinician needs to obtain different action pictures (e.g., a different boy eating pizza, a pizza that looks different from the original training stimulus, and so forth).* **Therefore, for each irregular past, three trials are provided on the recording sheet to probe three varieties of each stimulus.**

When the child fails to produce a generalized response, give additional training trials on the already trained exemplar. Alternate probes and treatment until the child gives the same trained response on three trials in sequence for each exemplar.

Scripts for Probe Trials

Clinician	[Presents an untrained stimulus] "What did the boy do yesterday? Start with *the boy*"	No modeling; only a prompt
Child	"The boy ate pizza yesterday."	A correct, generalized response
Clinician	Scores the response as correct.	Offers no reinforcement
Clinician	[Presents another untrained stimulus] "What did the girl do earlier? Start with *the girl . . .*"	The second probe trial
Child	"Broke toy."	A wrong probe response
Clinician	Scores the response as incorrect.	Offers no corrective feedback

Name:	Date:	Session #:		
Age:	**Clinician:**			
Disorder: Language	**Target: Irregular Past in Expanded Sentences (Probe)**			
Untrained Stimuli	**Score: + correct; – incorrect or no responses**			
Note: Only the stimulus is new or untrained	Trial 1	Trial 2	Trial 3	
1. [The] boy ate pizza yesterday. (UT)				
2. [The] girl broke the toy earlier. (UT)				
3. [The] baby fell down last night. (UT)				
4. [The] man caught the ball fast. (UT)				
5. She came home from work. (UT)				
6. [The] doggie swam in the cold pool. (UT)				
7. [The] girl found the ball in the box. (UT)				
8. [The] boy built a tall tower. (UT)				
9. [The] man slept on the sofa last night. (UT)				
10. [The] boy hid the car under the table. (UT)				
Percent correct probe (Critcrion: 90%)				

If the child does not meet the probe criterion, give additional training on the trained sentences, and sub-sequently, readminister the probe trials. When the child gives correct responses on three consecutive trials, consider that exemplar trained. Then, either teach other irregular past morphemes or shift train-ing to conversational speech in which the production of irregular past words are monitored and reinforced.

Regular Past *d*
Regular Past *d* in Phrases
Baserate Protocols

Administer the evoked trials first followed by modeled trials. Do not provide feedback on any trials; just record the responses on the recording sheet provided on the next page or printed from the CD.

Scripts for Evoked Baserate Trial		Note
Clinician	[showing the picture of a boy putting a letter in a mail box] "This boy just mailed a letter. What did the boy do?	No modeling
Child	"Mail letter."	A wrong response
Clinician	Records the response as incorrect.	No corrective feedback
Clinician	[showing the picture of a woman moving a chair across room] "She just moved the chair from here to there. What did she do?"	The next trial
Child	"She moved." ["She moved chair"]	A correct response
Clinician	Records the response as correct.	No verbal praise

Administer the modeled baserate trials only after completing the evoked trials on all 20 (or more) exemplars.

Scripts for Modeled Baserate Trial		Note
Clinician	[showing the picture of a boy putting a letter in a mail box] "This boy just mailed a letter. What did the boy do? Say, *mailed a letter*."	Modeling
Child	"Mail letter."	A wrong response
Clinician	Records the response as incorrect.	No corrective feedback
Clinician	[showing the picture of a woman moving a chair across the room] "She just moved the chair. What did she do?" Say, *moved the chair*."	Modeling
Child	"Moved chair." ["Moved the chair."]	A correct response; the article may be missing
Clinician	Records the response.	No verbal praise

Baserate at least 20 exemplars as shown on the next page.

Baserating Regular Past *d* in Phrases
Exemplars and Recording Sheet

Print this page from the CD or photocopy this page for your clinical use.

Name/Age:	Date:
Goal: To establish the baserates of regular past *d* in basic sentences when asked questions while showing a picture.	Clinician:

Clinician's Comments:

Scoring: Correct: ✓ Incorrect or no response: X

Regular Past *d* in Phrases	Evoked	Modeled
1. mailed a letter		
2. moved the chair		
3. dialed the number		
4. closed the door		
5. rained yesterday		
6. covered the gift		
7. played on grass		
8. combed hair		
9. climbed fence		
10. poured juice		
11. opened the box		
12. dried the pot		
13. pulled rope		
14. waved bye bye		
15. peeled apples		
16. boy sneezed		
17. man smelled		
18. spilled water		
19. Mother hugged		
20. girl changed		
Percent correct baserate		

After establishing the baserates, initiate treatment. Use the protocols that follow.

Regular Past *d* in Phrases
Treatment Protocols

Important: *Give a few modeled trials at the word level if the child has difficulty imitating sentences that contain the regular past* d *words. If needed, give a detailed background information. For example, give instructions like the following:*

> *"We will work on a few words that help you talk about what just happened or some time ago. See, in this picture, the boy just dropped a letter into this mailbox. He just mailed a letter. What did he do? Say, mailed."*

Such detailed background information may be repeated on a few initial trials and periodically given as found necessary. It may not be needed on every trial, however.

Scripts for Modeled Discrete Trial Training		Note
Clinician	[showing the picture of a boy putting a letter in a mailbox] "This boy just mailed a letter. What did the boy do? Say, *mailed a letter.*"	Vocal emphasis on the target morpheme
Child	"Mail letter."	A wrong response
Clinician	"No, that is not correct. The boy just mailed a letter. Say, *mailed a letter.*"	Corrective feedback; vocal emphasis on the target morpheme
Child	"Mailed a letter."	A correct response
Clinician	"Very good! You said *mailed a letter!*"	Verbal praise

Repeat the trials until the child gives 5 consecutively correct, imitated responses. When the child imitates 5 correct responses in sequence, fade the modeling. Always point to the target action before asking a question.

Scripts for Fading the Modeling		Note
Clinician	"The boy just mailed a letter. What did the boy do? Say, *mail . . .*"	Partial modeling only
Child	"Mail" ["The boy mail."]	A wrong response
Clinician	"No, that is not correct. The boy mailed a letter. Don't forget the *d*. What did the boy do? Say, *mail . . .*"	Corrective feedback and partial modeling
Child	"Mailed a letter."	A correct response
Clinician	"Very good! You said *mailed a letter!*"	Verbal praise
Clinician	"What did the boy do?"	**An Evoked Trial**
Child	"Mailed a letter." ["Boy mailed letter."]	Correct answer; the articles may be missing

If the wrong responses persist on 4 to 5 evoked trials, reinstate partial or full modeling for a few trials, again fade the modeling, and re-present the evoked trials.

When the child meets the tentative learning criterion of 10 consecutively correct, nonimitated responses for a given exemplar, move on to the next exemplar. With this procedure, teach 8 to 10 exemplars. Use different exemplars as you see fit for a given child. Use the exemplars and the recording sheet given on the next page (or copy it from the CD).

Regular Past *d* in Phrases

Exemplars and Treatment Recording Sheet

Print this page from the CD or photocopy this page for your clinical use.

Teach a set of functional exemplars using the previous scripts. To teach additional irregular plural words, print this page from CD and type in new exemplars (of the kind given on the Baserate Recording Sheet).

Name/Age:	Date:
Goal: Production of the regular past *d* in phrases with 90% accuracy when asked questions while showing pictures.	Clinician:

Clinician's Comments:

Scoring: Correct: ✓   Incorrect or no response: X

Target skills	Discrete Trials														
	1	2	3	4	5	6	7	8	9	10	11	12	13	14	15
1. mailed a letter															
2. moved the chair															
3. dialed the number															
4. closed the door															
5. rained yesterday															
6. covered the gift															
7. played on grass															
8. combed hair															
9. climbed fence															
10. poured juice															

Teach 8 to 10 exemplars each to a training criterion of 10 consecutively correct, nonimitated responses. Then, shift training to the sentence level. Before teaching the regular past words in sentences, baserate their productions.

Regular Past *d* in Sentences

Baserate Protocols

Present pictures as found appropriate.

Scripts for Evoked Baserate Trial		Note
Clinician	[showing the picture of a boy putting a letter in a mailbox] "This boy just mailed a letter. What did the boy do? Start with *the boy . . .*"	No modeling, but prompting the production of a sentence
Child	"The boy mail letter." ["Mail letter."]	A wrong response
Clinician	Records the response as incorrect.	No corrective feedback
Clinician	[showing the picture of a woman moving a chair across room] "She just moved the chair." What did she do? Start with *she . . .*"	The next trial
Child	"She moved chair." ["She moved the chair."]	A correct response; articles may be produced or not
Clinician	Records the response as correct.	No verbal praise

Administer the modeled baserate trials only after completing the evoked trials on all 20 (or more) exemplars.

Scripts for Modeled Baserate Trial		Note
Clinician	[showing the picture of a boy putting a letter in a mailbox] "This boy just mailed a letter. What did the boy do? Say, *the boy mailed a letter.*"	Modeling
Child	"Boy mail letter."	A wrong response
Clinician	Records the response as incorrect.	No corrective feedback
Clinician	[showing the picture of a woman moving a chair across room] "She just moved the chair." What did she do? Say, *she moved the chair.*"	Modeling
Child	"She moved the chair." ["She moved chair."]	A correct response; articles may be missing
Clinician	Records the response.	No verbal praise

Baserate at least 20 exemplars as shown on the next page.

Regular Past *d* in Sentences

Exemplars and Baserate Recording Sheet

Print this page from the CD or photocopy this page for your clinical use.

Unless previously taught, consider the production of the article in brackets as optional.

Name/Age:	Date:
Goal: To establish the baserates of regular past *d* in sentences when asked questions while showing a picture.	Clinician:

Clinician's Comments:

Scoring: Correct: ✓ Incorrect or no response: X

Regular Past *d* in Sentences	Evoked	Modeled
1. [The] boy mailed a letter.		
2. She moved [the] chair.		
3. He dialed [the] number.		
4. She closed [the] door.		
5. It rained yesterday.		
6. [The] boy covered the gift.		
7. They played on grass.		
8. [The] girl combed her hair.		
9. [The] boy climbed the fence.		
10. [The] girl poured some juice.		
11. [The] man opened the box.		
12. [The] boy dried [the] pot.		
13. [The] girl pulled [the] rope.		
14. [The] boy waved bye bye.		
15. [The] woman peeled some apples.		
16. [The] boy sneezed yesterday.		
17. [The] man smelled the roses.		
18. [The] girl spilled water.		
19. [The] mother hugged her baby.		
20. [The] girl changed her dress.		
Percent correct baserate		

After establishing the baserates for the target sentences, initiate treatment. Use the protocols given on the next page.

Regular Past *d* in Sentences

Treatment Protocols

Scripts for Modeled Discrete Trial Training		Note
Clinician	[showing the picture of a boy putting a letter in a mailbox] "This boy just mailed a letter. What did the boy do? Say, *the boy mailed a letter.*"	Vocal emphasis on the target feature
Child	"Mail letter." ["Boy mail letter."]	Scored as a wrong response
Clinician	"No, you forgot to add d to mail. What did the boy do? Say, the boy *mailed a letter.*"	Corrective feedback; vocal emphasis on the target feature
Child	"The boy mailed a letter."	Scored as correct; the article may be missing
Clinician	"Very good! You said the boy *mailed a letter!*"	Verbal praise

Repeat the trials until the child gives 5 consecutively correct, imitated responses. When the child imitates 5 correct responses in sequence, fade the modeling. Always point to the target action before asking a question.

Scripts for Fading the Modeling		Note
Clinician	[showing the picture of a boy putting a letter in a mailbox] "This boy just mailed a letter. What did the boy do? Say, *the boy . . .*"	Partial modeling only
Child	"Mailed letter."	A wrong response
Clinician	"No, you didn't say the whole sentence. What did the boy do? Say, *the boy . . .*"	Corrective feedback and partial modeling
Child	"The boy mailed a letter."	A correct response
Clinician	"Very good! You said, *the boy mailed a letter!*"	Verbal praise
Clinician	"What did the boy do?"	**An Evoked Trial**
Child	"The boy mailed a letter."	Correct answer
Clinician	"Excellent! You said the whole sentence!"	Verbal praise

Regular Past *d* in Sentences

Exemplars and Treatment Recording Sheet

Print this page from the CD or photocopy this page for your clinical use.

Name/Age:	Date:
Goal: Production of the regular past *d* in sentences with 90% accuracy when asked questions while showing pictures.	Clinician:

Clinician's Comments:

Scoring: Correct: ✓   Incorrect or no response: X

Target skills	Discrete Trials														
	1	2	3	4	5	6	7	8	9	10	11	12	13	14	15
1. [The] boy mailed a letter.															
2. She moved [the] chair.															
3. He dialed [the] number.															
4. She closed [the] door.															
5. It rained yesterday.															
6. [The] boy covered the gift.															
7. They played on grass.															
8. [The] girl combed her hair.															
9. [The] boy climbed the fence.															
10. [The] girl poured some juice.															

When the child has met the learning criterion of 10 consecutively correct, evoked (nonimitated) responses for each of the 10 target sentences, conduct a probe to see if the production of regular past d has generalized to untrained stimuli.

Use the protocols given on the next page (or print it from the CD).

Regular Past *d* in Sentences
Probe Protocols and Recording Sheet

Print this page from the CD or photocopy this page for your clinical use.

On the probes, present the untrained exemplars (UT). When the child fails to meet the 90% correct probe criterion, either teach 2 to 4 new exemplars or give additional training trials on already trained exemplars. If needed, select new exemplars for probes. Probe at least 10 untrained exemplars. Alternate probes and treatment until the probe criterion is met.

Scripts for Probe Trials

Clinician	[Presents an untrained stimulus] "What did the man do? Start with *the man* . . ."	No modeling; only a prompt
Child	"The man opened the box."	A correct, generalized response
Clinician	Scores the response as correct.	Offers no reinforcement
Clinician	[Presents another untrained stimulus] "What did the boy do? Start with *the boy* . . ."	The second probe trial
Child	"dried pot."	A wrong probe response
Clinician	Scores the response as incorrect.	Offers no corrective feedback

Name:	Date:	Session #:
Age:	**Clinician:**	
Disorder: Language	**Target: Regular past *d* in Sentences (Probe)**	

Untrained Stimuli	Score: + correct; – incorrect or no responses
1. [The] man opened [the] box. (UT)	
2. [The] boy dried [the] pot. (UT)	
3. [The] girl pulled [the] rope. (UT)	
4. [The] boy waved bye bye. (UT)	
5. [The] woman peeled some apples. (UT)	
6. [The] boy sneezed yesterday. (UT)	
7. [The] man smelled [the] roses. (UT)	
8. [The] girl spilled water. (UT)	
9. [The] mother hugged her baby. (UT)	
10. [The] girl changed her dress. (UT)	
Percent correct probe (Criterion: 90%)	

If the child does not meet the probe criterion, give additional training on the trained sentences, or teach new exemplars. Subsequently, readminister the probe trials. When the child meets 90% correct probe criterion, teach another morphologic feature or shift training to conversational speech in which the production of regular past d is monitored and reinforced.

Regular Past *t*
Regular Past *t* in Phrases
Baserate Protocols

Administer the evoked trials first followed by modeled trials. Do not provide feedback on any trials; just record the responses on the recording sheet provided on the next page or printed from the CD.

Scripts for Evoked Baserate Trial		Note
Clinician	[showing the picture of a girl walking toward her home] "The girl just walked from school to her home. What did the girl do?"	No modeling
Child	"Girl walk." ["Walk."]	A wrong response
Clinician	Records the response as incorrect.	No corrective feedback
Clinician	[showing the picture of a man next to a pile of raked leaves] "The man just raked all these leaves. What did the man do?"	The next trial
Child	"Man raked." ["Raked."]	A correct response
Clinician	Records the response as correct.	No verbal praise

Administer the modeled baserate trials only after completing the evoked trials on all 20 (or more) exemplars.

Scripts for Modeled Baserate Trial		Note
Clinician	[showing the picture of a girl walking toward her home] "The girl just walked from school to her home. What did the girl do?" Say, *the girl walked.*"	Modeling
Child	"Girl walk."	A wrong response
Clinician	Records the response as incorrect.	No corrective feedback
Clinician	[showing the picture of a man next to a pile of raked leaves] "The man just raked all these leaves. What did the man do? Say, *the man raked.*"	Modeling
Child	"Man raked." ["Man raked leaves."]	A correct response; an article may be missing
Clinician	Records the response.	No verbal praise

Baserate at least 20 exemplars as shown on the next page.

Regular Past *t* in Phrases

Exemplars and Baserate Recording Sheet

Print this page from the CD or photocopy this page for your clinical use.

Replace or add exemplars as you see fit to suit an individual child. Consider the production of the article in brackets as optional.

Name/Age:	Date:
Goal: To establish the baserates of regular past *t* words in phrases when asked questions while showing a picture.	Clinician:

Clinician's Comments:

Scoring: Correct: ✓   Incorrect or no response: X

Regular Past *t* in Phrases	Evoked	Modeled
1. [the] girl walked		
2. [the] man raked		
3. [the] woman baked		
4. [the] man fixed		
5. [the] boy brushed		
6. [the] girl picked		
7. [the] woman washed		
8. [the] man cooked		
9. [the] man dropped		
10. [the] boy kicked		
11. [the] girl pushed		
12. [the] boy bumped		
13. [the] girl crossed		
14. Grandma packed		
15. [the] boy zipped		
16. [the] lady sipped		
17. [the] dog splashed		
18. [the] girl licked		
19. [the] boy mopped		
20. [the girl] wiped		
Percent correct baserate		

After establishing the baserates, initiate treatment. Use the protocols that follow.

Regular Past *t* in Phrases

Treatment Protocols

Important: *Give a few modeled trials at the word level if the child has difficulty imitating sentences that contain the regular past* t *words. If needed, give a detailed background information. For example, give instructions like the following:*

> *"We will work on a few words that help you talk about what just happened sometime ago. See, in this picture, the man just raked all these leaves. What did he do? Say, raked."*

Such detailed background information may be repeated on a few initial trials and periodically given as found necessary. It may not be needed on every trial, however.

Scripts for Modeled Discrete Trial Training		Note
Clinician	[showing the picture of a girl walking toward her home] "The girl just walked from school to her home. What did the girl do?" Say, *the girl walked.*"	Vocal emphasis on the target morpheme
Child	"Girl walk." ["Walk."]	A wrong response
Clinician	"No, that is not correct. The girl just walked from school. Say, *girl walked.*"	Corrective feedback; vocal emphasis on the target morpheme
Child	"Girl walked." ["The girl walked."]	A correct response
Clinician	"Very good! You said girl **walked**!"	Verbal praise

Repeat the trials until the child gives 5 consecutively correct, imitated responses. When the child imitates 5 correct responses in sequence, fade the modeling. Always point to the target action before asking a question.

Scripts for Fading the Modeling		Note
Clinician	[showing the picture] "The girl just walked from school. What did the girl do? Say, *girl . . .*"	Partial modeling only
Child	"Walk" ["The girl walk."]	A wrong response
Clinician	"No, that is not correct. *The girl walked*. Don't forget the *t* at the end. What did the girl do? Say, *the girl . . .*"	Corrective feedback and partial modeling
Child	"Girl walked."	A correct response
Clinician	"Very good! You said *girl walked*!"	Verbal praise
Clinician	"What did the girl do?"	**An Evoked Trial**
Child	"Girl walked."	Correct answer; the articles may be missing

If the wrong responses persist on 4 to 5 evoked trials, reinstate partial or full modeling for a few trials, again fade the modeling, and re-present the evoked trials.

When the child meets the tentative learning criterion of 10 consecutively correct, nonimitated responses for a given exemplar, move on to the next exemplar. With this procedure, teach 8 to 10 exemplars. Use different exemplars as you see fit for a given child. Use the exemplars and the recording sheet given on the next page (or print it from the CD).

Regular Past *t* in Phrases

Exemplars and Treatment Recording Sheet

Print this page from the CD or photocopy this page for your clinical use.

Teach a set of functional exemplars using the previous scripts. To teach additional exemplars of regular past t *in sentences, print this page from CD and type in new exemplars (of the kind given on the Baserate Recording Sheet). Unless previously taught, consider the articles in brackets as optional.*

Name/Age:	Date:
Goal: Production of the regular past *t* words in phrases with 90% accuracy when asked questions while showing a picture.	Clinician:

Clinician's Comments:

Scoring: Correct: ✓ Incorrect or no response: X

Target skills	Discrete Trials														
	1	2	3	4	5	6	7	8	9	10	11	12	13	14	15
1. [the] girl walked															
2. [the] man raked															
3. [the] woman baked															
4. [the] man fixed															
5. [the] boy brushed															
6. [the] girl picked															
7. [the] woman washed															
8. [the] man cooked															
9. [the] man dropped															
10. [the] boy kicked															

Teach 8 to 10 exemplars each to a training criterion of 10 consecutively correct, nonimitated responses. Then, shift training to the sentence level. Before teaching the regular past t *words in sentences, baserate their productions. Use the protocols that follow.*

Regular Past *t* in Sentences

Baserate Protocols

On each trial, present an appropriate picture.

Scripts for Evoked Baserate Trial		Note
Clinician	[showing the picture of a girl walking toward her home] "The girl just walked from school to her home. What did the girl do?" Start with *the girl . . .*"	No modeling, but prompting the production of a sentence
Child	"The girl walk." ["Walk."]	A wrong response
Clinician	Records the response as incorrect.	No corrective feedback
Clinician	[showing the picture of a man next to a pile of raked leaves] "The man just raked all these leaves. What did the man do?" Start with *the man . . .*"	The next trial
Child	"The man raked leaves." ["Man raked leaves."]	A correct response; articles may be missing
Clinician	Records the response as correct.	No verbal praise

Administer the modeled baserate trials only after completing the evoked trials on all 20 (or more) exemplars.

Scripts for Modeled Baserate Trial		Note
Clinician	[showing the picture of a girl walking toward her home] "The girl just walked home from school. What did the girl do? Say, *the girl walked home.*"	Modeling
Child	"Girl walk home."	A wrong response
Clinician	Records the response as incorrect.	No corrective feedback
Clinician	[showing the picture of a man next to a pile of raked leaves] "The man just raked all these leaves. What did the man do? Say, *the man raked the leaves.*"	Modeling
Child	"The man raked the leaves."	A correct response; articles may be missing
Clinician	Records the response.	No verbal praise

Baserate at least 20 exemplars as shown on the next page.

Regular Past *t* in Sentences

Exemplars and Baserate Recording Sheet

Print this page from the CD or photocopy this page for your clinical use.

Name/Age:	Date:
Goal: To establish the baserates of regular past *t* words in sentences when asked questions while showing a picture.	Clinician:

Clinician's Comments:

Scoring: Correct: ✓   Incorrect or no response: X

Regular Past *t* in Sentences	Evoked	Modeled
1. [The] girl walked home.		
2. [The] man raked the leaves.		
3. [The] woman baked a cake.		
4. [The] man fixed the car.		
5. [The] boy brushed his teeth.		
6. [The] girl picked a flower.		
7. [The] woman washed her car.		
8. [The] man cooked a meal.		
9. [The] man dropped the plate.		
10. [The] boy kicked the ball.		
11. [The] girl pushed the table.		
12. [The] boy bumped the car.		
13. [The] girl crossed the street.		
14. Grandma packed the lunch.		
15. [The] boy zipped his jacket.		
16. [The] lady sipped her coffee.		
17. [The] dog splashed water.		
18. [The] girl licked ice cream.		
19. [The] boy mopped the floor.		
20. [The] girl wiped her tears.		
Percent correct baserate		

After establishing the baserates for the target sentences, initiate treatment. Use the protocols given on the next page.

Regular Past *t* in Sentences

Treatment Protocols

Scripts for Modeled Discrete Trial Training		Note
Clinician	[showing the picture of a girl walking toward her home] "The girl just walked home from school. What did the girl do? Say, *the girl walked home.*"	Vocal emphasis on the target morpheme
Child	"Girl walk home." ["Girl walk."]	Scored as a wrong response
Clinician	"No, you forgot to add *t* to *walk*. What did the girl do? Say, *the girl walked home.*"	Corrective feedback; vocal emphasis on the target morpheme
Child	"The girl walked home."	Scored as correct; the article may be missing
Clinician	"Very good! You said *the girl walked home!*"	Verbal praise

Repeat the trials until the child gives 5 consecutively correct, imitated responses. When the child imitates 5 correct responses in sequence, fade the modeling. Always point to the target object before asking a question.

Scripts for Fading the Modeling		Note
Clinician	[showing the picture of a girl walking toward her home] "The girl just walked home from school. What did the girl do? Say, *the girl . . .*"	Partial modeling only
Child	"Walked home."	A wrong response
Clinician	"No, you didn't say the whole sentence. What did the girl do? Say, *the girl . . .*"	Corrective feedback and partial modeling
Child	"The girl walked home."	A correct response
Clinician	"Very good! You said, *the girl walked home!*"	Verbal praise
Clinician	"What did the girl do?"	**An Evoked Trial**
Child	"The girl walked home."	Correct answer
Clinician	"Excellent! You said the whole sentence!"	Verbal praise

Regular Past *t* in Sentences

Exemplars and Treatment Recording Sheet

Print this page from the CD or photocopy this page for your clinical use.

Name/Age:	Date:
Goal: Production of the regular past *t* words in sentences with 90% accuracy when asked questions and while showing pictures.	Clinician:

Clinician's Comments:

Scoring: Correct: ✓   Incorrect or no response: X

Target skills	Discrete Trials														
	1	2	3	4	5	6	7	8	9	10	11	12	13	14	15
1. [The] girl walked home.															
2. [The] man raked the leaves.															
3. [The] woman baked a cake.															
4. [The] man fixed the car.															
5. [The] boy brushed his teeth.															
6. [The] girl picked a flower.															
7. [The] woman washed her car.															
8. [The] man cooked a meal.															
9. [The] man dropped the plate.															
10. [The] boy kicked the ball.															

When the child has met the learning criterion of 10 consecutively correct, evoked (nonimitated) responses for each of the 10 target sentences, conduct a probe to see if the production of regular past t has generalized to untrained stimuli.

Use the protocols given on the next page (or print it from the CD).

Regular Past *t* in Sentences

Probe Protocols and Recording Sheet

Print this page from the CD or photocopy this page for your clinical use.

On the probes, present the untrained exemplars (UT). When the child fails to meet the 90% correct probe criterion, either teach 2 to 4 new exemplars or give additional training trials on already trained exemplars. If needed, select new exemplars for probes. Probe at least 10 untrained exemplars. Alternate probes and treatment until the probe criterion is met.

Scripts for Probe Trials

Clinician	[Presents an untrained stimulus] "What did the girl do? Start with *the girl* . . . "	No modeling; only a prompt
Child	"The girl pushed the table."	A correct, generalized response
Clinician	Scores the response as correct.	Offers no reinforcement
Clinician	[Presents another untrained stimulus] "What did the boy do? Start with *the boy* . . . "	The second probe trial
Child	"Bump car."	A wrong probe response
Clinician	Scores the response as incorrect.	Offers no corrective feedback

Name:	Date:	Session #:
Age:	**Clinician:**	
Disorder: Language	**Target: Regular past *t* in Sentences (Probe)**	
Untrained Stimuli	**Score: + correct; – incorrect or no responses**	
1. [The] girl pushed the table. (UT)		
2. [The] boy bumped the car. (UT)		
3. [The] girl crossed the street. (UT)		
4. Grandma packed the lunch. (UT)		
5. [The] boy zipped his jacket. (UT)		
6. [The] lady sipped her coffee. (UT)		
7. [The] dog splashed water. (UT)		
8. [The] girl licked ice cream. (UT)		
9. [The] boy mopped the floor. (UT)		
10. [The] girl wiped her tears. (UT)		
Percent correct probe (Criterion: 90%)		

If the child does not meet the probe criterion, give additional training on the trained sentences, or teach new exemplars. Subsequently, readminister the probe trials. When the child meets 90% correct probe criterion, teach another morphologic feature or shift training to conversational speech in which the production of regular past t *is monitored and reinforced.*

Regular Past *ed*
Regular Past *ed* in Phrases

Baserate Protocols

Administer the evoked trials first followed by modeled trials. Do not provide feedback on any trials; just record the responses on the recording sheet provided on the next page or printed from the CD.

Scripts for Evoked Baserate Trial		Note
Clinician	[showing the picture of a woman folding a towel] "The woman just folded this towel. What did the woman do?"	No modeling
Child	"Fold towel." ["Fold."]	A wrong response
Clinician	Records the response as incorrect.	No corrective feedback
Clinician	[showing the picture of a man with a paint brush standing next to a freshly painted wall] "The man just painted this wall. What did the man do?"	The next trial
Child	"Man painted." ["Painted."]	A correct response
Clinician	Records the response as correct.	No verbal praise

Administer the modeled baserate trials only after completing the evoked trials on all 20 (or more) exemplars.

Scripts for Modeled Baserate Trial		Note
Clinician	[showing the picture of a woman folding a towel] "The woman just folded this towel. What did the woman do?" Say, *the woman folded.*"	Modeling
Child	"Woman fold." ["Fold"]	A wrong response
Clinician	Records the response as incorrect.	No corrective feedback
Clinician	[showing the picture of a man with a paint brush] "The man just painted. What did the man do?" Say, *the man painted.*"	Modeling
Child	"Man painted." ["The man painted."]	A correct response; articles may be missing
Clinician	Records the response.	No verbal praise

Baserate at least 20 exemplars as shown on the next page.

Regular Past *ed* in Phrases
Exemplars and Baserate Recording Sheet

Print this page from the CD or photocopy this page for your clinical use.

Replace or add exemplars as you see fit to suit an individual child. Consider the production of the article in brackets as optional.

Name/Age:	Date:
Goal: To establish the baserates of regular past *ed* words in phrases when asked questions while showing a picture.	Clinician:

Clinician's Comments:

Scoring: Correct: ✓ Incorrect or no response: X

Regular Past *ed* in Phrases	Evoked	Modeled
1. [the] woman folded		
2. [the] main painted		
3. [the] girl tasted		
4. [the] man skated		
5. ice cream melted		
6. she dusted		
7. [the] woman floated		
8. [the] woman knitted		
9. she tasted		
10. [the] girl rested		
11. they waited		
12. he saluted		
13. [the] boy pointed		
14. [the] girl potted		
15. [the] man pasted		
16. [the] boy counted		
17. he pointed		
18. she skated		
19. he bended		
20. the man planted		
Percent correct baserate		

After establishing the baserates, initiate treatment. Use the protocols that follow.

Regular Past *ed* in Phrases

Treatment Protocols

Important: *Give a few modeled trials at the word level if the child has difficulty imitating sentences that contain the regular past ed words. If needed, give a detailed background information. For example, give instructions like the following:*

> *"We will work on a few words that help you talk about what just happened or some time ago. See, in this picture, the woman just folded a towel. What did the woman do? Say, folded."*

Such detailed background information may be repeated on a few initial trials and periodically given as found necessary. It may not be needed on every trial, however.

Scripts for Modeled Discrete Trial Training		Note
Clinician	[showing the picture of a woman folding a towel] "The woman just folded this towel. What did the woman do?" Say, *the woman folded.*"	Vocal emphasis on the target morpheme
Child	"Woman fold." ["Fold."]	A wrong response
Clinician	"No, that is not correct. The woman just folded a towel. Say, *the woman fold**ed**.*"	Corrective feedback; vocal emphasis on the target morpheme
Child	"Woman folded." ["The woman folded."]	A correct response
Clinician	"Very good! You said, woman *fold**ed**!*"	Verbal praise

Repeat the trials until the child gives 5 consecutively correct, imitated responses. When the child imitates 5 correct responses in sequence, fade the modeling. Always point to the target object before asking a question.

Scripts for Fading the Modeling		Note
Clinician	[showing the picture of a woman folding a towel] "The woman just folded a towel. What did the woman do? Say, *the woman . . .*"	Partial modeling only
Child	"Fold" ["The woman fold."]	A wrong response
Clinician	"No, that is not correct. *The woman fold**ed**.* Don't forget the *ded* at the end. What did the woman do? Say, *the woman . . .*"	Corrective feedback and partial modeling
Child	"Woman folded." ["The woman folded."]	A correct response
Clinician	"Very good! You said, *woman fold**ed**!*"	Verbal praise
Clinician	"What did the woman do?"	**An Evoked Trial**
Child	"Woman folded."	Correct answer; the articles may be missing

If the wrong responses persist on 4 to 5 evoked trials, reinstate partial or full modeling for a few trials, again fade the modeling, and re-present the evoked trials.

When the child meets the tentative learning criterion of 10 consecutively correct, nonimitated responses for a given exemplar, move on to the next exemplar. With this procedure, teach 8 to 10 exemplars. Use different exemplars as you see fit for a given child. Use the exemplars and the recording sheet given on the next page (or print it from the CD).

Regular Past *ed* in Phrases

Exemplars and Treatment Recording Sheet

Print this page from the CD or photocopy this page for your clinical use.

Teach a set of functional exemplars using the previous scripts. To teach additional irregular plural words, print this page from CD and type in new exemplars (of the kind given on the Baserating Recording Sheet).

Name/Age:	Date:
Goal: Production of the regular past *ed* words in phrases with 90% accuracy.	Clinician:

Clinician's Comments:

Scoring: Correct: ✓   Incorrect or no response: X

Target skills	Discrete Trials														
	1	2	3	4	5	6	7	8	9	10	11	12	13	14	15
1. [the] woman folded															
2. [the] man painted															
3. [the] girl tasted															
4. [the] man skated															
5. ice cream melted															
6. she dusted															
7. [the] woman floated															
8. [the] woman knitted															
9. she tasted															
10. [the] girl rested															

Teach 8 to 10 exemplars each to a training criterion of 10 consecutively correct, nonimitated responses. Then, shift training to the sentence level. Before teaching the regular past words in sentences, base-rate their productions. Use the protocols that follow.

Regular Past *ed* in Sentences

Baserate Protocols

On each trial, present an appropriate picture.

Administer the evoked trials first, followed by modeled trials. Do not provide feedback on any trials; just record the child's responses on the recording sheet provided on the next page or printed from the CD.

Scripts for Evoked Baserate Trial		Note
Clinician	[showing the picture of a woman folding a towel] "The woman just folded this towel. What did the woman do?" Start with *the woman . . .*"	No modeling, but prompting the production of a sentence
Child	"The woman fold." ["Woman folded."]	A wrong response
Clinician	Records the response as incorrect.	No corrective feedback
Clinician	[showing the picture of a man with a paint brush standing next to a freshly painted wall] "The man just painted this wall. What did the man do? Start with *the man . . .*"	The next trial
Child	"The man painted." ["Man painted wall."]	A correct response; articles may be missing
Clinician	Records the response as correct.	No verbal praise

Administer the modeled baserate trials only after completing the evoked trials on all 20 (or more) exemplars.

Scripts for Modeled Baserate Trial		Note
Clinician	[showing the picture of a woman folding a towel] "The woman just folded this towel. What did the woman do?" Say, *the woman folded the towel.*"	Modeling
Child	"Woman folded."	A wrong response
Clinician	Records the response as incorrect.	No corrective feedback
Clinician	[showing the picture of a man with a paint brush standing next to a freshly painted wall] "The man just painted this wall. What did the man do?" Say, *the man painted the wall.*"	Modeling
Child	"The man painted the wall."	A correct response; article may be missing
Clinician	Records the response.	No verbal praise

Baserate at least 20 exemplars as shown on the next page.

Regular Past *ed* in Sentences

Exemplars and Baserate Recording Sheet

Print this page from the CD or photocopy this page for your clinical use.

Name/Age:	Date:
Goal: To establish the baserates of regular past *ed* words in sentences when asked questions while showing a picture.	Clinician:

Clinician's Comments:

Scoring: Correct: ✓   Incorrect or no response: X

Regular Past *ed* in Sentences	Evoked	Modeled
1. [The] woman folded the towel.		
2. [The] man painted the wall.		
3. [The] girl tasted the ice cream.		
4. [The] man skated on ice.		
5. Her ice cream melted.		
6. She dusted the table.		
7. [The] woman floated on water.		
8. [The] woman knitted a sweater.		
9. She tasted the food.		
10. [The] girl rested on the grass.		
11. They waited in the restaurant.		
12. He saluted the flag.		
13. [The] boy pointed to the picture.		
14. [The] girl potted a plant.		
15. [The] man pasted a sign.		
16. [The] boy counted the coins.		
17. He pointed to the cat.		
18. She skated on ice.		
19. He bended the wire.		
20. [The] man planted a tree.		
Percent correct baserate		

Replace or add new exemplars as you see fit for a given child.

After establishing the baserates for the target sentences, initiate treatment. Use the protocols given on the next page.

Regular Past *ed* in Sentences

Treatment Protocols

Scripts for Modeled Discrete Trial Training		Note
Clinician	[showing the picture of a woman folding a towel] "The woman just folded this towel. What did the woman do?" Say, *the woman fol**ded** the towel."*	Vocal emphasis on the target morpheme
Child	"Woman folded."	Scored as a wrong response
Clinician	"No, you said folded, which is good, but you forgot to say the whole sentence. What did the woman do? Say, *the woman fol**ded** the towel."*	Corrective feedback; vocal emphasis on the target morpheme
Child	"The woman folded the towel."	Scored as correct; the article may be missing
Clinician	"Very good! You said *the woman fol**ded** the towel!"*	Verbal praise

Repeat the trials until the child gives 5 consecutively correct, imitated responses. When the child imitates 5 correct responses in sequence, fade the modeling. Always point to the target object before asking a question.

Scripts for Fading the Modeling		Note
Clinician	[showing the picture of a woman folding a towel] "The woman just folded this towel. What did the woman do?" Say, *the woman . . ."*	Partial modeling only
Child	"Folded towel."	A wrong response
Clinician	"No, you didn't say the whole sentence. What did the woman do? Say, *the woman . . ."*	Corrective feedback and partial modeling
Child	"The woman folded the towel."	A correct response
Clinician	"Very good! You said, *the woman folded the towel!"*	Verbal praise
Clinician	"What did the woman do?"	**An Evoked Trial**
Child	"The woman folded the towel."	Correct answer
Clinician	"Excellent! You said the whole sentence!"	Verbal praise

Regular Past *ed* in Sentences

Exemplars and Treatment Recording Sheet

Print this page from the CD or photocopy this page for your clinical use.

Name/Age:	Date:
Goal: Production of the regular past *ed* words in sentences with 90% accuracy when asked questions while showing a picture.	Clinician:

Clinician's Comments:

Scoring: Correct: ✓   Incorrect or no response: X

Target skills	Discrete Trials														
	1	2	3	4	5	6	7	8	9	10	11	12	13	14	15
1. [The] woman folded the towel.															
2. [The] man painted the wall.															
3. [The] girl tasted the ice cream.															
4. [The] man skated on ice.															
5. Her ice cream melted.															
6. She dusted the table.															
7. [The] woman floated on water.															
8. [The] woman knitted a sweater.															
9. She tasted the food.															
10. [The] girl rested on the grass.															

When the child has met the learning criterion of 10 consecutively correct, evoked (nonimitated) responses for each of the 10 target sentences, conduct a probe to see if the production of regular past ed has generalized to untrained stimuli.

Use the protocols given on the next page (or print it from the CD).

Regular Past *ed* in Sentences

Probe Protocols and Recording Sheet

Print this page from the CD or photocopy this page for your clinical use.

On the probes, present the untrained exemplars (UT). When the child fails to meet the 90% correct probe criterion, either teach 2 to 4 new exemplars or give additional training trials on already trained exemplars. If needed, select new exemplars for probes. Probe at least 10 untrained exemplars. Alternate probes and treatment until the probe criterion is met.

Scripts for Probe Trials

Clinician	[Presents an untrained stimulus] "Before they were seated, they waited in the restaurant. What did they do at the restaurant? Start with *they* . . ."	No modeling; only a prompt
Child	"They waited in the restaurant."	A correct, generalized response
Clinician	Scores the response as correct.	Offers no reinforcement
Clinician	[Presents another untrained stimulus] "He just did something to the flag. What did he do? Start with *he* . . ."	The second probe trial
Child	"salute flag."	A wrong probe response
Clinician	Scores the response as incorrect.	Offers no corrective feedback

Name:	Date:		Session #:
Age:	**Clinician:**		
Disorder: Language	**Target: Regular past *ed* in Sentences (Probe)**		
Untrained Stimuli	**Score: + correct; – incorrect or no responses**		
1. They waited in the restaurant. (UT)			
2. He saluted the flag. (UT)			
3. [The] boy pointed to the picture. (UT)			
4. [The] girl potted a plant. (UT)			
5. [The] man pasted a sign. (UT)			
6. [The] boy counted the coins. (UT)			
7. He pointed to the cat. (UT)			
8. She skated on ice. (UT)			
9. He bended the wire. (UT)			
10. [The] man planted a tree. UT)			
Percent correct probe (Criterion: 90%)			

If the child does not meet the probe criterion, give additional training on the trained sentences, or teach new exemplars. Subsequently, readminister the probe trials. When the child meets 90% correct probe criterion, teach another morphologic feature or shift training to conversational speech in which the production of regular past ed *is monitored and reinforced.*

Pronouns

Overview

In sentences, pronouns replace nouns. Along with nouns and verbs, pronouns are essential elements of many sentences. Pronouns take different grammatical functions or forms. The same form of a pronoun may be classified differently depending on the grammatical function it serves in a sentence.

Personal pronouns are a large collection of independent target responses. They include:

> *he, she, it, I, me, we, us, my, mine, our, ours, you, your, yours, its, him, his, her, hers, they, them, their,* and *theirs*

Personal pronouns may be further classified into the subjective case (e.g., *he, she, it*), the objective case (e.g., *him, her, them*), and the possessive case (e.g., *my, his, her*).

Indefinite pronouns (e.g., *many, few*) reflexive pronouns (e.g., *myself, yourself, themselves*), interrogative pronouns (e.g., *who, which, that, whom, whose, whatever*), demonstrative pronouns (e.g., *this, that, these, those*), and reciprocal pronouns (e.g., *each other, one another*) are among the other kinds of English pronouns.

General Training Strategy

Children with language disorders often confuse pronouns; children with autism are especially prone to this confusion. Because pronouns help express various kinds of experiences in varied sentence forms, they are an important treatment target for most children with language disorders. Among the many forms of pronouns, *personal pronouns* are a functional early treatment target.

Most forms of pronouns are a large collection of independent response classes; all forms need to be taught because there would be no generalized production from one kind of pronoun learning to another kind. When the child has mastered a few functional personal pronouns, the clinician may consider teaching other forms of pronouns (e.g., the *indefinite* or the *relative*).

Protocols are provided for selected personal pronouns only. The same general strategy may be used to teach other forms of personal and other kinds of pronouns. Type in the new pronoun targets on the generic baserate, treatment, and probe recording sheets you will find on the CD and print them for clinical use.

Pronoun *he*
Pronoun *he* in Basic Sentences

Baserate Protocols

Administer the evoked trials first followed by modeled trials. Do not provide feedback on any trials; just record the child's responses on the recording sheet provided on the next page or printed from the CD.

Scripts for Evoked Baserate Trial		Note
Clinician	[showing the picture of a man playing a piano] "He plays the piano. Who plays the piano?"	No modeling
Child	"Plays piano." ["Piano."]	A wrong response
Clinician	Records the response as incorrect.	No corrective feedback
Clinician	[showing the picture of a man washing the dishes] "He washes dishes. Who washes the dishes?"	The next trial
Child	"He washes." ["He washes dishes."]	A correct response
Clinician	Records the response as correct.	No verbal praise

Administer the modeled baserate trials only after completing the evoked trials on all 20 (or more) exemplars.

Scripts for Modeled Baserate Trial		Note
Clinician	[showing the picture of a man playing a piano] "He plays the piano. Who plays the piano? Say, *he plays the piano.*"	Modeling
Child	"Play piano." ["Plays piano"]	A wrong response
Clinician	Records the response as incorrect.	No corrective feedback
Clinician	[showing the picture of a man washing the dishes] "He washes dishes. Who washes the dishes? Say, *he washes the dishes.*"	Modeling
Child	"He washes the dishes." ["He washes dishes."]	A correct response; article may be missing
Clinician	Records the response.	No verbal praise

Baserate at least 20 exemplars as shown on the next page.

Pronoun *he* in Basic Sentences

Exemplars and Baserate Recording Sheet

Print this page from the CD or photocopy this page for your clinical use.

Name/Age:	Date:
Goal: To establish the baserates of pronoun *he* in basic sentences when asked questions while showing a picture.	Clinician:

Clinician's Comments:

Scoring: Correct: ✓ Incorrect or no response: X

Pronoun *he* in Basic Sentences	Evoked	Modeled
1. He plays.		
2. He washes.		
3. He walks.		
4. He kicks.		
5. He eats.		
6. He digs.		
7. He runs.		
8. He talks.		
9. He cries.		
10. He smiles.		
11. He dances.		
12. He sings.		
13. He marches.		
14. He reads.		
15. He builds.		
16. He bowls.		
17. He sleeps.		
18. He writes.		
19. He opens.		
20. He pushes.		
Percent correct baserate		

After establishing the baserates, initiate treatment. Use the protocols that follow.

Pronoun *he* in Basic Sentences

Treatment Protocols

Scripts for Modeled Discrete Trial Training		Note
Clinician	[showing the picture of a man playing a piano] "He plays the piano. Who plays the piano? Say, **he** *plays the piano*."	Vocal emphasis on the target morpheme
Child	"Play piano." ["Piano."]	A wrong response
Clinician	"No, that is not correct. He plays piano. Say, **he** *plays piano*."	Corrective feedback; vocal emphasis on the pronoun
Child	"He plays piano." ["He plays the piano."]	A correct response
Clinician	"Very good! You said, he *plays piano!*"	Verbal praise

Repeat the trials until the child gives 5 consecutively correct, imitated responses. When the child imitates 5 correct responses in sequence, fade the modeling. Always point to the target object before asking a question.

Scripts for Fading the Modeling		Note
Clinician	[showing the picture of a man playing a piano] "He plays the piano. Who plays the piano? Say, *he . . .* "	Partial modeling only
Child	"Plays piano."	A wrong response
Clinician	"No, that is not correct. **He** *plays the piano.* Don't forget the *he* at the beginning. Who plays the piano? Say, *he . . .* "	Corrective feedback and partial modeling
Child	"He plays the piano." ["He plays piano."]	A correct response
Clinician	"Very good! You said, *he plays piano!*"	Verbal praise
Clinician	"Who plays the piano?"	**An Evoked Trial**
Child	"He plays the piano."	Correct answer; the articles may be missing

If the wrong responses persist on 4 to 5 evoked trials, reinstate partial or full modeling for a few trials, again fade the modeling, and re-present the evoked trials.

When the child meets the tentative learning criterion of 10 consecutively correct, nonimitated responses for a given exemplar, move on to the next exemplar. With this procedure, teach 8 to 10 exemplars. Use different exemplars as you see fit for a given child. Use the exemplars and the recording sheet given on the next page (or print it from the CD).

Pronoun *he* in Basic Sentences

Exemplars and Treatment Recording Sheet

Print this page from the CD or photocopy this page for your clinical use.

Teach a set of functional exemplars using the previous scripts. To teach additional exemplars with the pronoun he, *print this page from the CD and type in new exemplars (of the kind given on the Baserate Recording Sheet).*

Name/Age:	Date:
Goal: Production of pronoun *he* in basic sentences with 90% accuracy when asked questions while showing a picture.	Clinician:

Clinician's Comments:

Scoring: Correct: ✓   Incorrect or no response: X

Target skills	Discrete Trials														
	1	2	3	4	5	6	7	8	9	10	11	12	13	14	15
1. He plays.															
2. He washes.															
3. He walks.															
4. He kicks.															
5. He eats.															
6. He digs.															
7. He runs.															
8. He talks.															
9. He cries.															
10. He smiles.															

Teach 8 to 10 exemplars each to a training criterion of 10 consecutively correct nonimitated responses. Then, shift training to the expanded sentence level. Before teaching the pronoun he *in expanded sentences, baserate their productions. Use the protocols that follow.*

Pronoun *he* in Expanded Sentences

Baserate Protocols

Scripts for Evoked Baserate Trial		Note
Clinician	[showing the picture of a man playing a piano] "He plays the piano. Who plays the piano?"	No modeling
Child	"Man plays." ["Plays piano."]	A wrong response
Clinician	Records the response as incorrect.	No corrective feedback
Clinician	[showing the picture of a man washing dishes] "He washes the dishes. Who washes the dishes?"	The next trial
Child	"He washes dishes." ["He washes."]	A correct response; articles may be missing
Clinician	Records the response as correct.	No verbal praise

Administer the modeled baserate trials only after completing the evoked trials on all 20 (or more) exemplars.

Scripts for Modeled Baserate Trial		Note
Clinician	[showing the picture of a man playing a piano] "He plays the piano. Who plays the piano? Say, *he plays the piano.*"	Modeling
Child	"Plays the piano."	A wrong response
Clinician	Records the response as incorrect.	No corrective feedback
Clinician	[showing the picture of a man washing dishes] "He washes the dishes. Who washes the dishes? Say, *he washes the dishes.*"	Modeling
Child	"He washes the dishes."	A correct response; article may be missing
Clinician	Records the response.	No verbal praise

Baserate at least 20 exemplars as shown on the next page.

Pronoun *he* in Expanded Sentences

Exemplars and Baserate Recording Sheet

Print this page from the CD or photocopy this page for your clinical use.

Name/Age:	Date:
Goal: To establish the baserates of pronoun *he* in expanded sentences when asked questions while showing a picture.	Clinician:

Clinician's Comments:

Scoring: Correct: ✓   Incorrect or no response: X

Pronoun *he* in Expanded Sentences	Evoked	Modeled
1. He plays the piano.		
2. He washes the dishes.		
3. He walks home.		
4. He kicks the ball.		
5. He eats a sandwich.		
6. He digs a hole.		
7. He runs to the store.		
8. He talks to the lady.		
9. He cries in the school.		
10. He smiles at the baby.		
11. He dances on the floor.		
12. He sings on the stage.		
13. He marches on the grass.		
14. He reads a book.		
15. He builds a house.		
16. He bowls in a bowling alley.		
17. He sleeps on the sofa.		
18. He writes a letter.		
19. He opens the box.		
20. He pushes a cart.		
Percent correct baserate		

After establishing the baserates for the target sentences, initiate treatment. Use the protocols given on the next page.

Pronoun *he* in Expanded Sentences
Treatment Protocols

Scripts for Modeled Discrete Trial Training		Note
Clinician	[showing the picture of a man playing a piano] "He plays the piano. Who plays the piano? Say, **he** *plays the piano.*"	Vocal emphasis on the target word
Child	"Plays piano." ["Man plays piano."]	Scored as a wrong response
Clinician	"No, you forgot **he**. Who plays the piano? Say, **he** *plays the piano.*"	Corrective feedback; vocal emphasis on the target word
Child	"He plays the piano." ["He plays piano."]	Scored as correct; the article may be missing
Clinician	"Very good! You said, **he** *plays the piano!*"	Verbal praise

Repeat the trials until the child gives 5 consecutively correct, imitated responses. When the child imitates 5 correct responses in sequence, fade the modeling.

Scripts for Fading the Modeling		Note
Clinician	[showing the picture of a man playing a piano] "He plays the piano. Who plays the piano? Say, **he** . . ."	Partial modeling only
Child	"Plays piano."	A wrong response
Clinician	"No, you didn't start with **he**. Who plays the piano? Say, *he* . . ."	Corrective feedback and partial modeling
Child	"He plays the piano."	A correct response; article may be missing
Clinician	"Very good! You said, **he** *plays the piano!*"	Verbal praise
Clinician	"Who plays the piano?"	**An Evoked Trial**
Child	"He plays the piano."	Correct answer
Clinician	"Excellent! You said the whole sentence!"	Verbal praise

Pronoun *he* in Expanded Sentences

Exemplars and Treatment Recording Sheet

Print this page from the CD or photocopy this page for your clinical use.

Name/Age:	Date:
Goal: Production of pronoun *he* in expanded sentences with 90% accuracy when asked questions while showing a picture.	Clinician:

Clinician's Comments:

Scoring: Correct: ✓   Incorrect or no response: X

Target skills	Discrete Trials														
	1	2	3	4	5	6	7	8	9	10	11	12	13	14	15
1. He plays the piano.															
2. He washes the dishes.															
3. He walks home.															
4. He kicks the ball.															
5. He eats a sandwich.															
6. He digs a hole.															
7. He runs to the store.															
8. He talks to the lady.															
9. He cries in the school.															
10. He smiles at the baby.															

When the child has met the learning criterion of 10 consecutively correct, evoked (nonimitated) responses for each of the 10 target sentences, conduct a probe to see if the production of the pronoun has generalized to untrained stimuli. Use the probe protocols given on the next page (or print it from the CD).

Pronoun *he* in Expanded Sentences
Probe Protocols and Recording Sheet

Print this page from the CD or photocopy this page for your clinical use.

On the probes, present the untrained exemplars (UT). When the child fails to meet the 90% correct probe criterion, either teach 2 to 4 new exemplars or give additional training trials on already trained exemplars. If needed, select new exemplars for probes. Probe at least 10 untrained exemplars. Alternate probes and treatment until the probe criterion is met.

Scripts for Probe Trials

Clinician	[Presents an untrained stimulus] "This man dances on the floor. Who dances on the floor? Start with *he . . .*"	No modeling; only a prompt
Child	"He dances on the floor." ["He dances on floor."]	A correct, generalized response
Clinician	Scores the response as correct.	Offers no reinforcement
Clinician	[Presents another untrained stimulus] "He sings on the stage. Who sings on the stage? Start with *he . . .*"	The second probe trial
Child	"Sings." ["Sings on stage."]	A wrong probe response
Clinician	Scores the response as incorrect.	Offers no corrective feedback

Name:	Date:	Session #:
Age:	Clinician:	
Disorder: Language	**Target: Pronoun *he* in expanded sentences (Probe)**	

Untrained Stimuli	Score: + correct; – incorrect or no responses
1. He dances on the floor.	
2. He sings on the stage.	
3. He marches on the grass.	
4. He reads a book.	
5. He builds a house.	
6. He bowls in a bowling alley.	
7. He sleeps on the sofa.	
8. He writes a letter.	
9. He opens the box.	
10. He pushes a cart.	
Percent correct probe (Criterion: 90%)	

If the child does not meet the probe criterion, give additional training on the trained sentences, or teach new exemplars. Subsequently, readminister the probe trials. When the child meets 90% correct probe criterion, teach another morphologic feature or shift training to conversational speech in which the production of the pronoun is monitored and reinforced.

Pronoun *she*
Pronoun *she* in Phrases

Baserate Protocols

Administer the evoked trials first followed by modeled trials. Do not provide feedback on any trials; just record the responses on the recording sheet provided on the next page or printed from the CD.

Scripts for Evoked Baserate Trial		Note
Clinician	[showing the picture of a woman picking roses] "She picks the roses. Who picks the roses?"	No modeling
Child	"Pick roses." ["Picks roses."]	A wrong response
Clinician	Records the response as incorrect.	No corrective feedback
Clinician	[showing the picture of a woman mowing the lawn] "She mows the lawn. Who mows the lawn?"	The next trial
Child	"She mows." [She mows lawn."]	A correct response; article may be missing
Clinician	Records the response as correct.	No verbal praise

Administer the modeled baserate trials only after completing the evoked trials on all 20 (or more) exemplars.

Scripts for Modeled Baserate Trial		Note
Clinician	[showing the picture] "She picks the roses. Who picks the roses? Say, *she picks.*"	Modeling
Child	"Picks." ["Picks roses."]	A wrong response
Clinician	Records the response as incorrect.	No corrective feedback
Clinician	[showing the picture of a woman mowing the lawn] "She mows the lawn. Who mows the lawn? Say, *she mows.*"	Modeling
Child	"She mows."	A correct response; articles may be missing
Clinician	Records the response.	No verbal praise

Baserate at least 20 exemplars as shown on the next page.

Pronoun *she* in Phrases

Exemplars and Baserate Recording Sheet

Print this page from the CD or photocopy this page for your clinical use.

Name/Age:	Date:
Goal: To establish the baserates of pronoun *she* in phrases when asked questions while showing a picture.	Clinician:

Clinician's Comments:

Scoring: Correct: ✓   Incorrect or no response: X

Pronoun *she* in Phrases	Evoked	Modeled
1. She picks.		
2. She mows.		
3. She holds.		
4. She knits.		
5. She washes.		
6. She bakes.		
7. She walks.		
8. She rides.		
9. She drives.		
10. She cooks.		
11. She feeds.		
12. She throws.		
13. She lifts.		
14. She plays.		
15. She jumps.		
16. She combs.		
17. She plants.		
18. She teaches.		
19. She paints.		
20. She buys.		
Percent correct baserate		

After establishing the baserates, initiate treatment. Use the protocols that follow.

Pronoun *she* in Phrases

Treatment Protocols

Scripts for Modeled Discrete Trial Training		Note
Clinician	[showing the picture of a woman picking roses] "She picks the roses. Who picks the roses? Say, **she** *picks*."	Vocal emphasis on the target pronoun
Child	"Picks." ["Picks roses."]	A wrong response
Clinician	"No, that is not correct. Who picks the roses? Say, **she** *picks*."	Corrective feedback; vocal emphasis on the target pronoun
Child	"She picks." ["She picks roses."]	A correct response
Clinician	"Very good! You said, *she picks*!"	Verbal praise

Repeat the trials until the child gives 5 consecutively correct, imitated responses. When the child imitates 5 correct responses in sequence, fade the modeling. Always point to the target person before asking a question.

Scripts for Fading the Modeling		Note
Clinician	[showing the picture of a woman picking roses] "She picks the roses. Who picks the roses? Say, *she . . .*"	Partial modeling only
Child	"Picks roses" ["Picks the roses."]	A wrong response
Clinician	"No, that is not correct. **She** *picks the roses*. Don't forget the *she* at the beginning. Who picks the roses? Say, *she . . .*"	Corrective feedback and partial modeling
Child	"She picks . . ." ["She picks roses."]	A correct response
Clinician	"Very good! You said, *she picks*!"	Verbal praise
Clinician	"Who picks the roses?"	**An Evoked Trial**
Child	"She picks." ["She picks the roses."]	Correct answer; the articles may be missing

If the wrong responses persist on 4 to 5 evoked trials, reinstate partial or full modeling for a few trials, again fade the modeling, and re-present the evoked trials.

When the child meets the tentative learning criterion of 10 consecutively correct, nonimitated responses for a given exemplar, move on to the next exemplar. With this procedure, teach 8 to 10 exemplars. Use different exemplars as you see fit for a given child. Use the exemplars and the recording sheet given on the next page (or print it from the CD).

Pronoun *she* in Phrases

Exemplars and Treatment Recording Sheet

Print this page from the CD or photocopy this page for your clinical use.

Name/Age:	Date:
Goal: Production of pronoun *she* in phrases with 90% accuracy when asked questions while showing a picture.	Clinician:

Clinician's Comments:

Scoring: Correct: ✓   Incorrect or no response: X

Target skills	Discrete Trials														
	1	2	3	4	5	6	7	8	9	10	11	12	13	14	15
1. She picks.															
2. She mows.															
3. She holds.															
4. She knits.															
5. She washes.															
6. She bakes.															
7. She walks.															
8. She rides.															
9. She drives.															
10. She cooks.															

Teach 8 to 10 exemplars each to a training criterion of 10 consecutively correct, nonimitated responses. Then, shift training to sentences. Before teaching the pronoun in sentences, baserate their productions. Use the protocols that follow.

Pronoun *she* in Sentences

Baserate Protocols

Scripts for Evoked Baserate Trial		Note
Clinician	[showing the picture of a woman picking roses] "She picks the roses. Who picks the roses?"	No modeling
Child	"Picks roses."	A wrong response
Clinician	Records the response as incorrect.	No corrective feedback
Clinician	[showing the picture of a woman mowing the lawn] "She mows the lawn. Who mows the lawn?"	The next trial
Child	"She mows the lawn." ["She mows lawn."]	A correct response; articles may be missing
Clinician	Records the response as correct.	No verbal praise

Administer the modeled baserate trials only after completing the evoked trials on all 20 (or more) exemplars.

Scripts for Modeled Baserate Trial		Note
Clinician	[showing the picture of a woman picking the roses] "She picks the roses. Who picks the roses? Say, *she picks the roses.*"	Modeling
Child	"She picks." ["Picks roses."]	A wrong response
Clinician	Records the response as incorrect.	No corrective feedback
Clinician	[showing the picture of a woman mowing the lawn] "She mows the lawn. Who mows the lawn? Say, *she mows the lawn.*"	Modeling
Child	"She mows the lawn."	A correct response; the article may be missing
Clinician	Records the response.	No verbal praise

Baserate at least 20 exemplars as shown on the next page.

Pronoun *she* in Sentences

Exemplars and Baserate Recording Sheet

Print this page from the CD or photocopy this page for your clinical use.

Name/Age:	Date:
Goal: To establish the baserates of pronoun *she* in sentences when asked questions while showing a picture.	Clinician:

Clinician's Comments:

Scoring: Correct: ✓   Incorrect or no response: X

Pronoun *she* in Sentences	Evoked	Modeled
1. She picks the roses.		
2. She mows the lawn.		
3. She holds the candy.		
4. She knits the socks.		
5. She washes her face.		
6. She bakes cookies.		
7. She walks the doggie.		
8. She rides a bike.		
9. She drives a car.		
10. She cooks in the kitchen.		
11. She feeds the kitty.		
12. She throws a ball.		
13. She lifts the boxes.		
14. She plays a guitar.		
15. She jumps rope.		
16. She combs her hair.		
17. She plants flowers.		
18. She teaches in school.		
19. She paints a picture.		
20. She buys a toy.		
Percent correct baserate		

Replace or add new exemplars as you see fit for a given child.

After establishing the baserates for the target sentences, initiate treatment. Use the protocols given on the next page.

Pronoun *she* in Sentences

Treatment Protocols

Scripts for Modeled Discrete Trial Training		Note
Clinician	[showing the picture of a woman picking the roses] "She picks the roses. Who picks the roses? Say, **she** *picks the roses*."	Vocal emphasis on the target word
Child	"She picks." ["Picks the roses."]	Scored as a wrong response
Clinician	"No, you forgot **she**. What does she do? Say, **she** *picks the roses*."	Corrective feedback; vocal emphasis on the target word
Child	"She picks the roses." ["She picks roses."]	Scored as correct; the article may be missing
Clinician	"Very good! You said **she** *picks the roses*!"	Verbal praise

Repeat the trials until the child gives 5 consecutively correct, imitated responses. When the child imitates 5 correct responses in sequence, fade the modeling.

Scripts for Fading the Modeling		Note
Clinician	[showing the picture of a woman picking the roses] "She picks the roses. Who picks the roses? Say, **she** . . . "	Partial modeling only
Child	"Picks the roses."	A wrong response
Clinician	"No, you didn't start with **she**. What does she do? Say, *she* . . . "	Corrective feedback and partial modeling
Child	"She picks the roses."	A correct response; article may be missing.
Clinician	"Very good! You said, **she** *picks the roses*!"	Verbal praise
Clinician	"Who picks the roses?"	**An Evoked Trial**
Child	"She picks the roses."	Correct answer
Clinician	"Excellent! You said the whole sentence!"	Verbal praise

Pronoun *she* in Sentences

Exemplars and Treatment Recording Sheet

Print this page from the CD or photocopy this page for your clinical use.

Name/Age:	Date:
Goal: Production of pronoun *she* in sentences with 90% accuracy when asked questions while showing a picture.	Clinician:

Clinician's Comments:

Scoring: Correct: ✓   Incorrect or no response: X

Target skills	Discrete Trials														
	1	2	3	4	5	6	7	8	9	10	11	12	13	14	15
1. She picks the roses.															
2. She mows the grass.															
3. She holds the candy.															
4. She knits the socks.															
5. She washes her face.															
6. She bakes cookies.															
7. She walks the doggie.															
8. She rides a bike.															
9. She drives a car.															
10. She cooks in the kitchen.															

When the child has met the learning criterion of 10 consecutively correct, evoked (nonimitated) responses for each of the 10 target sentences, conduct a probe to see if the production of the pronoun has generalized to untrained stimuli. Use the probe protocols given on the next page (or print it from the CD).

Pronoun *she* in Sentences

Probe Protocols and Recording Sheet

Print this page from the CD or photocopy this page for your clinical use.

On the probes, present the untrained exemplars (UT). When the child fails to meet the 90% correct probe criterion, either teach 2 to 4 new exemplars or give additional training trials on already trained exemplars. If needed, select new exemplars for probes. Probe at least 10 untrained exemplars. Alternate probes and treatment until the probe criterion is met.

Scripts for Probe Trials

Clinician	[Presents an untrained stimulus] "She feeds the kitty. Who feeds the kitty? Start with *she* . . ."	No modeling; only a prompt
Child	"She feeds the kitty." ["She feeds kitty."]	A correct, generalized response
Clinician	Scores the response as correct.	Offers no reinforcement
Clinician	[Presents another untrained stimulus] "She throws a ball. Who throws a ball? Start with *she* . . ."	The second probe trial
Child	"Throws." ["Throws ball."]	A wrong probe response
Clinician	Scores the response as incorrect.	Offers no corrective feedback

Name:	Date:	Session #:
Age:	**Clinician:**	
Disorder: Language	**Target: Pronoun *she* in sentences (Probe)**	
Untrained Stimuli	**Score: + correct; – incorrect or no responses**	
1. She feeds the kitty. (UT)		
2. She throws a ball. (UT)		
3. She lifts the boxes. (UT)		
4. She plays a guitar. (UT)		
5. She jumps rope. (UT)		
6. She combs her hair. (UT)		
7. She plants flowers. (UT)		
8. She teaches in school. (UT)		
9. She paints a picture. (UT)		
10. She buys a toy. (UT)		
Percent correct probe		

If the child does not meet the probe criterion, give additional training on the trained sentences or teach new exemplars. Subsequently, readminister the probe trials. When the child meets 90% correct probe criterion, teach another morphologic feature or shift training to conversational speech in which the production of the pronoun is monitored and reinforced.

Pronoun *it*
Pronoun *it* in Phrases
Baserate Protocols

Administer the evoked trials first followed by modeled trials. Do not provide feedback on any trials; just record the child's responses on the recording sheet provided on the next page or printed from the CD

Scripts for Evoked Baserate Trial		Note
Clinician	[showing the picture of a bug crawling on the floor] "It crawls. What crawls?"	No modeling
Child	"Crawls."	A wrong response
Clinician	Records the response as incorrect.	No corrective feedback
Clinician	[showing the picture of a turtle moving] "It moves. What moves?"	The next trial
Child	"It moves."	A correct response
Clinician	Records the response as correct.	No verbal praise

Administer the modeled baserate trials only after completing the evoked trials on all 20 (or more) exemplars.

Scripts for Modeled Baserate Trial		Note
Clinician	[showing the picture of a bug crawling on the floor] "It crawls. What crawls? Say, *it crawls.*"	Modeling
Child	"Crawls."	A wrong response
Clinician	Records the response as incorrect.	No corrective feedback
Clinician	[showing the picture of a turtle moving] "It moves. What moves? Say, *it moves.*"	Modeling
Child	"It moves."	A correct response
Clinician	Records the response.	No verbal praise

Baserate at least 20 exemplars as shown on the next page.

Pronoun *it* in Phrases

Exemplars and Baserate Recording Sheet

Print this page from the CD or photocopy this page for your clinical use.

Replace or add exemplars as you see fit to suit an individual child.

Name/Age:	Date:
Goal: To establish the baserates of pronoun *it* in phrases when asked questions while showing a picture.	Clinician:

Clinician's Comments:

Scoring: Correct: ✓   Incorrect or no response: X

Pronoun *it* in Phrases	Evoked	Modeled
1. it crawls		
2. it moves		
3. it builds		
4. it washes		
5. it licks		
6. it kicks		
7. it runs		
8. it jumps		
9. it shows		
10. it eats		
11. it flies		
12. it lifts		
13. it rolls		
14. it chews		
15. it swims		
16. it feeds		
17. it barks		
18. it runs		
19. it sleeps		
20. it climbs		
Percent correct baserate		

After establishing the baserates, initiate treatment. Use the protocols given on the next page.

Teaching the Pronoun *it* in Phrases

Treatment Protocols

Scripts for Modeled Discrete Trial Training		Note
Clinician	[showing the picture of a bug crawling on the floor] "It crawls. What crawls? Say, *it crawls.*"	Vocal emphasis on the target morpheme
Child	"Crawls."	A wrong response
Clinician	"No, that is not correct. *It crawls.* What crawls?"	Corrective feedback; vocal emphasis on the pronoun
Child	"It crawls."	A correct response
Clinician	"Very good! You said, *it crawls!*"	Verbal praise

Repeat the trials until the child gives 5 consecutively correct, imitated responses. When the child imitates 5 correct responses in sequence, fade the modeling. Always point to the target stimulus before asking a question.

Scripts for Fading the Modeling		Note
Clinician	[showing the picture of a bug crawling on the floor] "It crawls. What crawls? Say, *it . . .*"	Partial modeling only
Child	"Crawls"	A wrong response
Clinician	"No, that is not correct. *It crawls.* Don't forget the *it* at the beginning. What does it do? Say, *It . . .*"	Corrective feedback and partial modeling
Child	"It crawls."	A correct response
Clinician	"Very good! You said, *it crawls!*"	Verbal praise
Clinician	"What crawls?"	**An Evoked Trial**
Child	"It crawls."	Correct answer; the articles may be missing

If the wrong responses persist on 4 to 5 evoked trials, reinstate partial or full modeling for a few trials, again fade the modeling, and re-present the evoked trials.

When the child meets the tentative learning criterion of 10 consecutively correct, nonimitated responses for a given exemplar, move on to the next exemplar. With this procedure, teach 8 to 10 exemplars. Use different exemplars as you see fit for a given child. Use the exemplars and the recording sheet given on the next page (or print it from the CD).

Pronoun *it* in Phrases

Exemplars and Treatment Recording Sheet

Print this page from the CD or photocopy this page for your clinical use.

Teach a set of functional exemplars using the previous scripts. To teach additional pronouns, print this page from CD and type in new exemplars (of the kind given on the Baserate Recording Sheet).

Name/Age:	Date:
Goal: Production of pronoun *it* in phrases with 90% accuracy when asked questions while showing a picture.	Clinician:

Clinician's Comments:

Scoring: Correct: ✓   Incorrect or no response: X

Target skills	Discrete Trials														
	1	2	3	4	5	6	7	8	9	10	11	12	13	14	15
1. it crawls															
2. it moves															
3. it builds															
4. it washes															
5. it licks															
6. it kicks															
7. it runs															
8. it jumps															
9. it shows															
10. it eats															

Teach 8 to 10 exemplars each to a training criterion of 10 consecutively correct, nonimitated responses. Then, shift training to the sentence level. Before teaching the pronoun in sentences, baserate their productions. Use the protocols that follow.

Pronoun *it* in Sentences
Baserate Protocols

Scripts for Evoked Baserate Trial		Note
Clinician	[showing the picture of a bug crawling on the floor] "It crawls on the floor. What crawls on the floor?"	No modeling
Child	"It crawls." ["Crawls on floor."]	A wrong response
Clinician	Records the response as incorrect.	No corrective feedback
Clinician	[showing the picture of a turtle moving] "It moves slowly. What moves slowly?"	The next trial
Child	"It moves slowly."	A correct response
Clinician	Records the response as correct.	No verbal praise

Administer the modeled baserate trials only after completing the evoked trials on all 20 (or more) exemplars.

Scripts for Modeled Baserate Trial		Note
Clinician	[showing the picture of a bug crawling on the floor] "It crawls on the floor. What crawls on the floor? Say, *it crawls on the floor.*"	Modeling
Child	"It crawls."	A wrong response
Clinician	Records the response as incorrect.	No corrective feedback
Clinician	[showing the picture of a turtle moving] "It moves slowly. What moves slowly? Say, *it moves slowly.*"	Modeling
Child	"It moves slowly."	A correct response
Clinician	Records the response.	No verbal praise

Baserate at least 20 exemplars as shown on the next page.

Pronoun *it* in Sentences

Exemplars and Baserate Recording Sheet

Print this page from the CD or photocopy this page for your clinical use.

Name/Age:	Date:
Goal: To establish the baserates of pronoun *it* in sentences when asked questions while showing a picture.	Clinician:

Clinician's Comments:

Scoring: Correct: ✓   Incorrect or no response: X

Pronoun *it* in Sentences	Evoked	Modeled
1. It crawls on the floor.		
2. It moves slowly.		
3. It builds a nest.		
4. It washes the dishes.		
5. It licks its paw.		
6. It kicks hard.		
7. It runs fast.		
8. It jumps high.		
9. It shows its teeth.		
10. It eats hay.		
11. It flies in the sky.		
12. It lifts the house.		
13. It rolls down the hill.		
14. It chews food.		
15. It swims in the pond.		
16. It feeds the baby		
17. It barks at the man.		
18. It runs to the cave.		
19. It sleeps in the bed.		
20. It climbs a tree.		
Percent correct baserate		

After establishing the baserates for the target sentences, initiate treatment. Use the protocols given on the next page.

Pronoun *it* in Sentences

Treatment Protocols

Scripts for Modeled Discrete Trial Training		Note
Clinician	[showing the picture of a bug crawling on the floor] "It crawls on the floor What crawls on the floor? Say, *it crawls on the floor*."	Vocal emphasis on the target word
Child	"It crawls. ["Crawls on the floor."]	Scored as a wrong response
Clinician	"No, you forgot *it*. What crawls on the floor? Say, *it crawls on the floor*."	Corrective feedback; vocal emphasis on the target words
Child	"It crawls on the floor." ["It crawls on floor."]	Scored as correct; the article may be missing
Clinician	"Very good! You said *it crawls on the floor*!"	Verbal praise

Repeat the trials until the child gives 5 consecutively correct, imitated responses. When the child imitates 5 correct responses in sequence, fade the modeling.

Scripts for Fading the Modeling		Note
Clinician	[showing the picture of a bug crawling on the floor] "It crawls on the floor. What crawls on the floor? Say, *it . . .* "	Partial modeling only
Child	"Crawls on floor."	A wrong response
Clinician	"No, you didn't start with *it*. What crawls on the floor? Say, *it . . .* "	Corrective feedback and partial modeling
Child	"It crawls on the floor."	A correct response; article may be missing.
Clinician	"Very good! You said, *it crawls on the floor*!"	Verbal praise
Clinician	"What crawls on the floor?"	**An Evoked Trial**
Child	"It crawls on the floor."	Correct answer
Clinician	"Excellent! You said the whole sentence!"	Verbal praise

Pronoun *it* in Sentences

Exemplars and Treatment Recording Sheet

Print this page from the CD or photocopy this page for your clinical use.

Name/Age:	Date:
Goal: Production of pronoun *it* in sentences with 90% accuracy when asked questions while showing a picture.	Clinician:

Clinician's Comments:

Scoring: Correct: ✓   Incorrect or no response: X

Target skills	Discrete Trials														
	1	2	3	4	5	6	7	8	9	10	11	12	13	14	15
1. It crawls on the floor.															
2. It moves slowly.															
3. It builds a nest.															
4. It washes the dishes.															
5. It licks its paw.															
6. It kicks hard.															
7. It runs fast.															
8. It jumps high.															
9. It shows its teeth.															
10. It eats hay.															

When the child has met the learning criterion of 10 consecutively correct, evoked (nonimitated) responses for each of the 10 target sentences, conduct a probe to see if the production of the pronoun has generalized to untrained stimuli. Use the probe protocols given on the next page (or print it from the CD).

Pronoun *it* in Sentences

Probe Protocols and Recording Sheet

Print this page from the CD or photocopy this page for your clinical use.

On the probes, present the untrained exemplars (UT). When the child fails to meet the 90% correct probe criterion, either teach 2 to 4 new exemplars or give additional training trials on already trained exemplars. If needed, select new exemplars for probes. Probe at least 10 untrained exemplars. Alternate probes and treatment until the probe criterion is met.

Scripts for Probe Trials

Clinician	[Presents an untrained stimulus] "It flies in the sky. What flies in the sky? Start with *it* . . ."	No modeling; only a prompt
Child	"It flies in the sky." ["It flies in sky."]	A correct, generalized response; article may be missing
Clinician	Scores the response as correct.	Offers no reinforcement
Clinician	[Presents another untrained stimulus] "It lifts the house. What lifts the house? Start with *it* . . ."	The second probe trial
Child	"Lifts." ["Lifts house."]	A wrong probe response
Clinician	Scores the response as incorrect.	Offers no corrective feedback

Name:	Date:	Session #:
Age:	Clinician:	
Disorder: Language	Target: Pronoun *it* in Sentences (Probe)	

Untrained Stimuli	Score: + correct; – incorrect or no responses
1. It flies in the sky.	
2. It lifts the house.	
3. It rolls down the hill.	
4. It chews food.	
5. It swims in the pond.	
6. It feeds the baby.	
7. It barks at the man.	
8. It runs to the cave.	
9. It sleeps in the bed.	
10. It climbs a tree.	
Percent correct probe (Criterion: 90%)	

If the child does not meet the probe criterion, give additional training on the trained sentences, or teach new exemplars. Subsequently, readminister the probe trials. When the child meets 90% correct probe criterion, teach another morphologic feature or shift training to conversational speech in which the production of the pronoun is monitored and reinforced.

Articles

Overview

The English articles include *a, an, one, some, the,* and so forth. Articles specify the quantity of a noun or help point out a particular one in a class or series. Of the five articles, *a, an, one,* and *some* are indefinite; *the* is definite. Roughly, when something is referred to the first time in speech or writing, the article *a* (or *an*) may be appropriate (e.g., "I saw *a* car pass by"). In subsequent references, the definite article *the* is appropriate ("*The* car that passed by was a Chevy"). Articles are essential for specificity in communication.

Brown's (1973) study ranked articles *a* and *the* as the eighth grammatical morpheme to meet the mastery criterion. As with other grammatic forms, children achieve mastery in producing articles at widely differing ages.

General Training Strategy

Children with language disorders have particular difficulty learning the correct production of articles. They are essential treatment targets. Articles are perhaps appropriately taught when the child's language skills have improved with successful teaching of other morphologic features, phrases, and simple sentences that are more functional than the articles.

Articles are more abstract than nouns, verbs, and adjectives. Although reciting the rules for their correct production may not be effective in teaching the articles to young children with language impairment, providing some general description of the conditions under which the articles are produced may be essential to orient them to the task. Teaching multiple and varied exemplars may be the most effective strategy.

Frequent probes to assess generalized production may be necessary to conclude that the child has learned to produce the articles correctly. The clinician may need to find additional exemplars for articles to teach children with language disorders. The clinician may type the new exemplars on the generic baserate, treatment, and probe recording sheets found on the CD.

Article *a*
Article *a* in Phrases
Baserate Protocols

Administer the evoked trials first followed by modeled trials. Do not provide feedback on any trials; just record the child's responses on the recording sheet provided on the next page or printed from the CD.

Because the articles are not obvious targets to the child, it may be helpful to orient the child to the target behavior on the few initial trials as the scripts make it clear. For instance, while showing the appropriate picture, the clinician may give additional information:

> *"When you are talking about only one animal, you add **a** to the word. For example, here you see only one dog. Therefore, you say, I see **a** dog. Here you see one chair. So you say, I see **a** chair. In this picture, you see one boy. You say, I see **a** boy."*

The clinician may illustrate a few such exemplars before initiating the formal baserate trials. On the base rate trials themselves, the clinician may refrain from offering such background information.

Scripts for Evoked Baserate Trial		Note
Clinician	[showing the picture of a dog] "What do you see?"	No modeling
Child	"Dog"	A wrong response
Clinician	Records the response as incorrect.	No corrective feedback
Clinician	[showing the picture of a kitten] "What do you see?"	The next trial
Child	"A kitty."	A correct response
Clinician	Records the response as correct.	No verbal praise

Administer the modeled baserate trials only after completing the evoked trials on all 20 (or more) exemplars.

Scripts for Modeled Baserate Trial		Note
Clinician	[showing the picture of a dog] "What do you see? Say, *a dog.*"	Modeling
Child	"Dog."	A wrong response
Clinician	Records the response as incorrect.	No corrective feedback
Clinician	[showing the picture of a kitten] "What do you see? Say, *a kitty.*"	Modeling
Child	"A kitty."	A correct response
Clinician	Records the response.	No verbal praise

Baserate at least 20 exemplars as shown on the next page.

Article *a* in Phrases

Exemplars and Baserate Recording Sheet

Print this page from the CD or photocopy this page for your clinical use.

Replace or add exemplars as you see fit to suit an individual child.

Name/Age:	Date:
Goal: To establish the baserates of article *a* in phrases when asked questions while showing a picture.	Clinician:

Clinician's Comments:

Scoring: Correct: ✓   Incorrect or no response: X

Article *a* in Phrases	Evoked	Modeled
1. a dog		
2. a kitty		
3. a lion		
4. a fish		
5. a bug		
6. a chair		
7. a plane		
8. a bird		
9. a truck		
10. a cup		
11. a kangaroo		
12. a clown		
13. a flower		
14. a sheep		
15. a boy		
16. a car		
17. a doll		
18. a woman		
19. a baby		
20. a man		
Percent correct baserate		

After establishing the baserates, initiate treatment. Use the protocols given on the next page.

Article *a* in Phrases

Treatment Protocols

Scripts for Modeled Discrete Trial Training		Note
Clinician	[showing the picture of a dog] "What do you see? Say, *a dog*."	Vocal emphasis on the target morpheme
Child	"Dog."	A wrong response
Clinician	"No, that is not correct; *a dog*. What do you see?"	Corrective feedback; vocal emphasis on the article
Child	"A dog."	A correct response
Clinician	"Very good! You said, *a dog*!"	Verbal praise

Repeat the trials until the child gives 5 consecutively correct, imitated responses. When the child imitates 5 correct responses in sequence, fade the modeling. Always point to the target object before asking a question.

Scripts for Fading the Modeling		Note
Clinician	[showing the picture of a kitten] "What do you see? Say, *a* . . . "	Partial modeling only
Child	"Kitty."	A wrong response
Clinician	"No, that is not correct; *a kitty*. Don't forget the *a* at the beginning. What do you see? Say, *a* . . . "	Corrective feedback and partial modeling
Child	"A kitty."	A correct response
Clinician	"Very good! You said, *a kitty*!"	Verbal praise
Clinician	"What do you see?"	**An Evoked Trial**
Child	"A kitty."	Correct answer

If the wrong responses persist on 4 to 5 evoked trials, reinstate partial or full modeling for a few trials, again fade the modeling, and re-present the evoked trials.

When the child meets the tentative learning criterion of 10 consecutively correct, nonimitated responses for a given exemplar, move on to the next exemplar. With this procedure, teach 8 to 10 exemplars. Use different exemplars as you see fit for a given child. Use the exemplars and the recording sheet given on the next page (or copy it from the CD).

Article *a* in Phrases

Exemplars and Treatment Recording Sheet

Print this page from the CD or photocopy this page for your clinical use.

Name/Age:	Date:
Goal: Production of the article *a* in phrases with 90% accuracy when asked questions while showing a picture.	Clinician:

Clinician's Comments:

Scoring: Correct: ✓   Incorrect or no response: X

Target skills	Discrete Trials														
	1	2	3	4	5	6	7	8	9	10	11	12	13	14	15
1. a dog															
2. a kitty															
3. a lion															
4. a fish															
5. a bug															
6. a chair															
7. a plane															
8. a bird															
9. a truck															
10. a cup															

Teach 8 to 10 exemplars each to a training criterion of 10 consecutively correct, nonimitated responses. Then, shift training to the sentence level. Before teaching the article in sentences, baserate their productions. Use the protocols that follow.

Article *a* in Sentences

Baserate Protocols

Scripts for Evoked Baserate Trial		Note
Clinician	[showing the picture of a dog] "What do you see? Start with *I see . . .*"	No modeling
Child	"A dog."	A wrong response
Clinician	Records the response as incorrect.	No corrective feedback
Clinician	[showing the picture of a kitten] "What do you see? Start with *I see . . .*"	The next trial
Child	"I see a dog."	A correct response
Clinician	Records the response as correct.	No verbal praise

Administer the modeled baserate trials only after completing the evoked trials on all 20 (or more) exemplars.

Scripts for Modeled Baserate Trial		Note
Clinician	[showing the picture of a dog] "What do you see? Say, *I see a dog.*"	Modeling
Child	"A dog."	A wrong response
Clinician	Records the response as incorrect.	No corrective feedback
Clinician	[showing the picture of a kitten] "What do you see? Say, *I see a kitty.*"	Modeling
Child	"I see a kitty."	A correct response
Clinician	Records the response.	No verbal praise

Baserate at least 20 exemplars as shown on the next page.

Article *a* in Sentences

Exemplars and Baserate Recording Sheet

Print this page from the CD or photocopy this page for your clinical use.

Name/Age:	Date:
Goal: To establish the baserates of the article *a* in sentences when asked questions while showing a picture.	Clinician:

Clinician's Comments:

Scoring: Correct: ✓   Incorrect or no response: X

Article *a* in Sentences	Evoked	Modeled
1. I see a dog.		
2. I see a kitty.		
3. I see a lion.		
4. I see a fish.		
5. I see a bug.		
6. I see a chair.		
7. I see a plane.		
8. I see a bird.		
9. I see a truck.		
10. I see a cup.		
11. I see s a kangaroo.		
12. I see a clown.		
13. I see a flower.		
14. I see a sheep.		
15. I see a boy.		
16. I see a car.		
17. I see a doll.		
18. I see a woman.		
19. I see a baby.		
20. I see a man.		
Percent correct baserate		

Replace or add new exemplars as you see fit for a given child.

After establishing the baserates for the target sentences, initiate treatment. Use the protocols given on the next page.

Article *a* in Sentences

Treatment Protocols

Scripts for Modeled Discrete Trial Training		Note
Clinician	[showing the picture of a dog] "What do you see? Say, *I see **a** dog.*"	Vocal emphasis on the target article
Child	"I see dog."	Scored as a wrong response
Clinician	"No, you forgot **a**. What do you see? Say, *I see **a** dog.*"	Corrective feedback; vocal emphasis on the article
Child	"I see a dog."	Scored as correct
Clinician	"Very good! You said, I see a dog!"	Verbal praise

Repeat the trials until the child gives 5 consecutively correct, imitated responses. When the child imitates 5 correct responses in sequence, fade the modeling.

Scripts for Fading the Modeling		Note
Clinician	[showing the picture of a dog] "What do you see? Say, *I see . . .*"	Partial modeling only
Child	"I see dog."	A wrong response
Clinician	"No, you forgot the **a**. What do you see? Say, *I see . . .*"	Corrective feedback and partial modeling
Child	"I see a dog."	A correct response
Clinician	"Very good! You said, I see **a** dog!"	Verbal praise
Clinician	"What do you see?"	**An Evoked Trial**
Child	"I see a dog."	Correct answer
Clinician	"Excellent! You said the whole sentence!"	Verbal praise

Article *a* in Sentences

Exemplars and Treatment Recording Sheet

Print this page from the CD or photocopy this page for your clinical use.

Name/Age:	Date:
Goal: Production of the article *a* in sentences with 90% accuracy when asked questions while showing a picture.	Clinician:

Clinician's Comments:

Scoring: Correct: ✓ Incorrect or no response: X

Target skills	Discrete Trials														
	1	2	3	4	5	6	7	8	9	10	11	12	13	14	15
1. I see a dog.															
2. I see a kitty.															
3. I see a lion.															
4. I see a fish.															
5. I see a bug.															
6. I see a chair.															
7. I see a plane.															
8. I see a bird.															
9. I see a truck.															
10. I see a cup.															

When the child has met the learning criterion of 10 consecutively correct, evoked (nonimitated) responses for each of the 10 target sentences, conduct a probe to see if the production of the article has generalized to untrained stimuli. Use the probe protocols given on the next page (or print it from the CD).

Article *a* in Sentences

Probe Protocols and Recording Sheet

Print this page from the CD or photocopy this page for your clinical use.

On the probes, present the untrained exemplars (UT). When the child fails to meet the 90% correct probe criterion, either teach 2 to 4 new exemplars or give additional training trials on already trained exemplars. If needed, select new exemplars for probes. Probe at least 10 untrained exemplars. Alternate probes and treatment until the probe criterion is met.

Scripts for Probe Trials

Clinician	[Presents an untrained stimulus] "What do you see? Start with *I see . . .*"	No modeling; only a prompt
Child	"I see a kangaroo."	A correct, generalized response
Clinician	Scores the response as correct.	Offers no reinforcement
Clinician	[Presents another untrained stimulus] "What do you see? Start with *I see . . .*"	The second probe trial
Child	"Clown."	A wrong probe response
Clinician	Scores the response as incorrect.	Offers no corrective feedback

Name:	Date:	Session #:
Age:	**Clinician:**	
Disorder: Language	**Target: Article *a* in Sentences (Probe)**	
Untrained Stimuli	**Score: + correct; – incorrect or no responses**	
1. I see a kangaroo. (UT)		
2. I see a clown. (UT)		
3. I see a flower. (UT)		
4. I see a sheep. (UT)		
5. I see a boy. (UT)		
6. I see a car. (UT)		
7. I see a doll. (UT)		
8. I see a woman. (UT)		
9. I see a baby. (UT)		
10. I see a man. (UT)		
Percent correct probe		

If the child does not meet the probe criterion, give additional training on the trained sentences or teach new exemplars. Subsequently, readminister the probe trials. When the child meets 90% correct probe criterion, teach another morphologic feature or shift training to conversational speech in which the production of the article is monitored and reinforced.

Article *the* in Phrases

Baserate Protocols

Administer the evoked trials first followed by modeled trials. Do not provide feedback on any trials; just record the responses on the recording sheet provided on the next page or printed from the CD.

Because the articles are not obvious targets to the child, it may be helpful to orient the child to the target behavior on the few initial trials as the scripts make it clear. Also, in teaching the definite article, **it may be helpful to use paired stimuli** *(e.g., a big elephant and a small ant). While showing such paired pictures, the clinician may give additional information:*

> *"When you are talking about something in particular, you add* the *to the word. For example, here you see a small ant and a big elephant. If someone asks, what is small? You say, the ant is small. Here you see a white puppy and a green frog. If someone asks you what is white? You say, the puppy is white. In this picture, you see a red ball and a yellow banana. If someone asks you what is red? You say,* **the** *ball is red."*

The clinician may illustrate a few such exemplars before initiating the formal baserate trials. On the baserate trials themselves, the clinician may refrain from offering such background information.

Scripts for Evoked Baserate Trial		Note
Clinician	[showing the picture of a small ant and a big elephant] "What is small?"	No modeling
Child	"Ant."	A wrong response
Clinician	Records the response as incorrect.	No corrective feedback
Clinician	[showing the picture of a white puppy and a green frog] "What is white?"	The next trial
Child	"The puppy."	A correct response
Clinician	Records the response as correct.	No verbal praise

Administer the modeled baserate trials only after completing the evoked trials on all 20 (or more) exemplars.

Scripts for Modeled Baserate Trial		Note
Clinician	[showing the picture of a small ant and a big elephant] "What is small? Say, *the ant.*"	Modeling
Child	"Ant."	A wrong response
Clinician	Records the response as incorrect.	No corrective feedback
Clinician	[showing the picture of a white puppy and a green frog] "What is white?" Say, *the puppy.*"	Modeling
Child	"The puppy."	A correct response
Clinician	Records the response.	No verbal praise

Baserate at least 20 exemplars as shown on the next page.

Article *the* in Phrases

Exemplars and Baserate Recording Sheet

Print this page from the CD or photocopy this page for your clinical use.

Replace or add exemplars as you see fit to suit an individual child.

Name/Age:	Date:
Goal: To establish the baserates of the article *the* in phrases when asked questions while showing a picture.	Clinician:

Clinician's Comments:

Scoring: Correct: ✓   Incorrect or no response: X

Article *the* in Phrases	Evoked	Modeled
1. the ant		
2. the puppy		
3. the ball		
4. the elephant		
5. the frog		
6. the banana		
7. the kite		
8. the book		
9. the doll		
10. the cookie		
11. the snake		
12. the tree		
13. the worm		
14. the apple		
15. the cup		
16. the sock		
17. the spoon		
18. the girl		
19. the baby		
20. the man		
Percent correct baserate		

After establishing the baserates, initiate treatment. Use the protocols given on the next page.

Article *the* in Phrases

Treatment Protocols

Scripts for Modeled Discrete Trial Training		Note
Clinician	[showing the picture of a small ant and a big elephant] "What is small? Say, **the** *ant*."	Vocal emphasis on the target morpheme
Child	"Ant."	A wrong response
Clinician	"No, that is not correct. **The** *ant*." What is small?"	Corrective feedback; vocal emphasis on the article
Child	"The ant."	A correct response
Clinician	"Very good! You said, *the ant!*"	Verbal praise

Repeat the trials until the child gives 5 consecutively correct, imitated responses. When the child imitates 5 correct responses in sequence, fade the modeling.

Scripts for Fading the Modeling		Note
Clinician	[showing the picture of a small ant and a big elephant] "What is small? Say, *the . . .*"	Partial modeling only
Child	"Ant"	A wrong response
Clinician	"No, that is not correct. **The** *ant*. Don't forget *the* at the beginning. What is small? Say, *the . . .*"	Corrective feedback and partial modeling
Child	"The ant."	A correct response
Clinician	"Very good! You said, *the ant!*"	Verbal praise
Clinician	"What is small?"	**An Evoked Trial**
Child	"The ant."	Correct answer

If the wrong responses persist on 4 to 5 evoked trials, reinstate partial or full modeling for a few trials, again fade the modeling, and re-present the evoked trials.

When the child meets the tentative learning criterion of 10 consecutively correct, nonimitated responses for a given exemplar, move on to the next exemplar. With this procedure, teach 8 to 10 exemplars. Use different exemplars as you see fit for a given child. Use the exemplars and the recording sheet given on the next page (or print it from the CD).

Article *the* in Phrases

Exemplars and Treatment Recording Sheet

Print this page from the CD or photocopy this page for your clinical use.

Name/Age:	Date:
Goal: Production of the article *the* in phrases with 90% accuracy when asked questions while showing a picture.	Clinician:

Clinician's Comments:

Scoring: Correct: ✓   Incorrect or no response: X

Target skills	Discrete Trials														
	1	2	3	4	5	6	7	8	9	10	11	12	13	14	15
1. the ant															
2. the puppy															
3. the ball															
4. the elephant															
5. the frog															
6. the banana															
7. the kite															
8. the book															
9. the doll															
10. the cookie															

Teach 8 to 10 exemplars each to a training criterion of 10 consecutively correct, nonimitated responses. Then, shift training to the sentence level. Before teaching the article in sentences, baserate their productions. Use the protocols that follow.

Article *the* in Sentences

Baserate Protocols

Scripts for Evoked Baserate Trial		Note
Clinician	[showing the picture of a small ant and a big elephant] "I want you to say the whole sentence this time. When I ask, what is small? you should say, *the ant is small*. So, what is small?"	No modeling but orienting the child to the expected response
Child	"The ant."	Scored as a wrong response
Clinician	Records the response as incorrect.	No corrective feedback
Clinician	[showing the picture of a white puppy and a green frog] "What is white?"	The next trial
Child	"The puppy is white."	A correct response
Clinician	Records the response as correct.	No verbal praise

Administer the modeled baserate trials only after completing the evoked trials on all 20 (or more) exemplars.

Scripts for Modeled Baserate Trial		Note
Clinician	[showing the picture of a small ant and a big elephant] "What is small?" Say, *the ant is small*."	Modeling
Child	"Ant is small."	A wrong response
Clinician	Records the response as incorrect.	No corrective feedback
Clinician	[showing the picture of a white puppy and a green frog] "What is white?" Say, *the puppy is white*."	Modeling
Child	"The puppy is white."	A correct response
Clinician	Records the response.	No verbal praise

Baserate at least 20 exemplars as shown on the next page.

Article *the* in Sentences

Exemplars and Baserate Recording Sheet

Print this page from the CD or photocopy this page for your clinical use.

Name/Age:	Date:
Goal: To establish the baserates of the article *the* in sentences when asked questions while showing a picture.	Clinician:

Clinician's Comments:

Scoring: Correct: ✓   Incorrect or no response: X

Article *the* in Sentences	Evoked	Modeled
1. The ant is small.		
2. The puppy is white.		
3. The ball is red.		
4. The elephant is big.		
5. The frog is jumping.		
6. The banana is yellow.		
7. The kite is flying.		
8. The book is thick.		
9. The doll is pretty.		
10. The cookie is round.		
11. The snake is long.		
12. The tree is tall.		
13. The worm is tiny.		
14. The apple is green.		
15. The cup is blue.		
16. The sock is dirty.		
17. The spoon is shiny.		
18. The girl is eating.		
19. The baby is smiling.		
20. The man is walking.		
Percent correct baserate		

Replace or add new exemplars as you see fit for a given child.

After establishing the baserates for the target sentences, initiate treatment. Use the protocols given on the next page.

Article *the* in Sentences

Treatment Protocols

Scripts for Modeled Discrete Trial Training		Note
Clinician	[showing the picture of a small ant and a big elephant] "What is small?" Say, ***the*** *ant is small.*"	Vocal emphasis on the target article
Child	"Ant is small."	Scored as a wrong response
Clinician	"No, you forgot ***the***. What is small? Say, ***the*** *ant is small.*"	Corrective feedback; vocal emphasis on the target article
Child	"The ant is small."	Scored as correct
Clinician	"Very good! You said, the ant is small!"	Verbal praise

Repeat the trials until the child gives 5 consecutively correct, imitated responses. When the child imitates 5 correct responses in sequence, fade the modeling.

Scripts for Fading the Modeling		Note
Clinician	[showing the picture of a small ant and a big elephant] "What is small? Say, *the . . .* "	Partial modeling only
Child	"Ant is small."	A wrong response
Clinician	"No, you forgot the. What is small? Say, *the . . .* "	Corrective feedback and partial modeling
Child	"The ant is small."	A correct response
Clinician	"Very good! You said, ***the*** ant is small!"	Verbal praise
Clinician	"What is small?"	**An Evoked Trial**
Child	"The ant is small."	Correct answer
Clinician	"Excellent! You said the whole sentence!"	Verbal praise

Article *the* in Sentences

Exemplars and Treatment Recording Sheet

Print this page from the CD or photocopy this page for your clinical use.

Name/Age:	Date:
Goal: Production of article *the* in sentences with 90% accuracy when asked questions while showing a picture.	Clinician:

Clinician's Comments:

Scoring: Correct: ✓ Incorrect or no response: X

Target skills	Discrete Trials														
	1	2	3	4	5	6	7	8	9	10	11	12	13	14	15
1. The ant is small.															
2. The puppy is white.															
3. The ball is red.															
4. The elephant is big.															
5. The frog is jumping.															
6. The banana is yellow.															
7. The kite is flying.															
8. The book is thick.															
9. The doll is pretty.															
10. The cookie is round.															

When the child has met the learning criterion of 10 consecutively correct, evoked (nonimitated) responses for each of the 10 target sentences, conduct a probe to see if the production of the article has generalized to untrained stimuli. Use the probe protocols given on the next page (or print it from the CD).

Article *the* in Sentences

Probe Protocols and Recording Sheet

Print this page from the CD or photocopy this page for your clinical use.

On the probes, present the untrained exemplars (UT). When the child fails to meet the 90% correct probe criterion, either teach 2 to 4 new exemplars or give additional training trials on already trained exemplars. If needed, select new exemplars for probes. Probe at least 10 untrained exemplars. Alternate probes and treatment until the probe criterion is met.

Scripts for Probe Trials

Clinician	[Presents a paired untrained stimulus: a short rope and a long snake] "The snake is long. What is long? Start with *the* . . . "	No modeling; only a prompt
Child	"The snake is long."	A correct, generalized response
Clinician	Scores the response as correct.	Offers no reinforcement
Clinician	[Presents another untrained stimulus pair: a short plant and a tall tree] "What is tall? Start with *the* . . . "	The second probe trial
Child	"Tree."	A wrong probe response
Clinician	Scores the response as incorrect.	Offers no corrective feedback

Name:	Date:	Session #:
Age:	**Clinician:**	
Disorder: Language	**Target: Article *the* in sentences (Probe)**	
Untrained Stimuli	**Score: + correct; – incorrect or no responses**	
1. The snake is long. (UT)		
2. The tree is tall. (UT)		
3. The worm is tiny. (UT)		
4. The apple is green. (UT)		
5. The cup is blue. (UT)		
6. The sock is dirty. (UT)		
7. The spoon is shiny. (UT)		
8. The girl is eating. (UT)		
9. The baby is smiling. (UT)		
10. The man is walking. (UT)		
Percent correct probe (Criterion: 90%)		

If the child does not meet the probe criterion, give additional training on the trained sentences, or teach new exemplars. Subsequently, readminister the probe trials. When the child meets 90% correct probe criterion, teach another morphologic feature or shift training to conversational speech in which the production of the article is monitored and reinforced.

Conjunctions

Overview

A **conjunction** is a grammatic morpheme that helps join or connect words, phrases, and sentences. Sentences that include conjunctions are more extended (in some cases more complex) than those without one or more conjunctions. Conjunctions in English may be coordinating, correlative, or subordinating.

Coordinating conjunctions *and, are,* and *but* join elements that are not identical but are of equal weight or value (as in *man* and *woman*). *And, but,* and *or* are the most frequently used coordinating conjunction in English (Hargis, 1977; Streng, 1972).

Correlative conjunctions also link elements of equal weight but are always used in pairs. They include *both . . . and, neither . . . nor,* and *either . . . or.* Finally, the varied English **subordinating conjunctions** connect an independent clause with an adverbial clause. They include, among others, *since, because, although, if, after, when, while, before, unless,* and so forth. There are other ways of classifying conjunctions. Some are classified as *conditional* (e.g., *if*), others as *causal* (e.g., *because, so, therefore*), and still others as *temporal* (e.g., *before, after, when, then*).

Brown's (1973) classic study on morphologic acquisition did not include conjunctions. Generally, preschool children begin to combine clauses with conjunctions. Improved narrative skills require the production of conjunctions. Up to 80% of the narratives school-age children produce may begin with the conjunction *and* (Hulit & Howard, 2002). In subsequent years, the conjunction *and* initiates progressively fewer narratives.

General Training Strategy

To learn the correct production of conjunctions, children should have mastered some basic phrases and sentences. Such mastery will make it easier for children to learn the correct production of conjunctions. They may be taught to combine what they already produce reliably.

It may be necessary to teach some conjunctions in phrases before moving on to grammatical clauses and sentences. Other conjunctions (e.g., *but*) need to be taught in sentences only. Such conjunctions as *and, but, or, because, if, before,* and *after* may be especially useful initial targets. Clinicians who choose conjunctions for which protocols are not provided may type them in on the generic baserate and treatment recording sheets provided on the CD.

Conjunction *and*
Conjunction *and* in Phrases
Baserate Protocols

Administer the evoked trials first followed by modeled trials. Do not provide feedback on any trials; just record the responses on the recording sheet provided on the next page or printed from the CD.

*Because the target conjunction may not be obvious to the child, it may be helpful to orient the child to the target behavior on the few initial trials. Also, in teaching the conjunction and, **it may be helpful to use paired stimuli** (e.g., a picture of milk and cookies, lions and tigers). While showing such paired pictures, the clinician may give additional information:*

> *"When you are talking about two or more things, you add the word **and** in between them. For example, in this picture, you see a glass of milk **and** some cookies. If someone asks, what do you see here? You say, I see milk **and** cookies. Here you see lions and tigers. If someone asks you what two animals do you see here? You say, lions **and** tigers."*

The clinician may illustrate a few such exemplars before initiating the formal baserate trials. On the baserate trials themselves, the clinician may refrain from offering such background information.

Scripts for Evoked Baserate Trial		Note
Clinician	[showing the paired picture of milk and cookies] "What two things do you see?"	No modeling
Child	"Milk." ["Cookies."]	A wrong response
Clinician	Records the response as incorrect.	No corrective feedback
Clinician	[showing the paired picture of a lion and a tiger] "What two animals do you see?"	The next trial
Child	"A lion and a tiger."	A correct response
Clinician	Records the response as correct.	No verbal praise

Administer the modeled baserate trials only after completing the evoked trials on all 20 (or more) exemplars.

Scripts for Modeled Baserate Trial		Note
Clinician	[showing the paired picture of milk and cookies] "What two things do you see? Say, *milk and cookies*."	Modeling
Child	"Cookies." ["Milk."]	A wrong response
Clinician	Records the response as incorrect.	No corrective feedback
Clinician	[showing the paired picture of lions and tigers] "What two animals do you see?" Say, *a lion and a tiger*."	Modeling
Child	"A lion and a tiger."	A correct response
Clinician	Records the response.	No verbal praise

Baserate at least 20 exemplars as shown on the next page.

Conjunction *and* in Phrases

Exemplars and Baserate Recording Sheet

Print this page from the CD or photocopy this page for your clinical use.

Replace or add exemplars as you see fit to suit an individual child.

Name/Age:	Date:
Goal: To establish the baserates of conjunction *and* in phrases when asked questions while showing a picture.	Clinician:

Clinician's Comments:

Scoring: Correct: ✓   Incorrect or no response: X

Conjunction *and* in Phrases	Evoked	Modeled
1. milk and cookie		
2. a lion and a tiger		
3. paper and pencil		
4. man and woman		
5. table and chair		
6. spoons and forks		
7. cars and trucks		
8. boys and girls		
9. worms and ants		
10. pie and pizza		
11. cups and plates		
12. hats and balloons		
13. bears and lions		
14. shoes and socks		
15. trains and planes		
16. pants and shirts		
17. fruits and vegetables		
18. baby and mother		
19. ball and bat		
20. cow and calf		
Percent correct baserate		

After establishing the baserates, initiate treatment. Use the protocols given on the next page.

Conjunction *and* in Phrases

Treatment Protocol

Scripts for Modeled Discrete Trial Training		Note
Clinician	[showing the paired picture of milk and cookies] "What two things do you see? Say, *milk **and** cookies*."	Vocal emphasis on the target morpheme
Child	"Milk." ["Cookies."]	A wrong response
Clinician	"No, that is not correct. Milk **and** *cookies*." What two things do you see? Say, *milk **and** cookies*."	Corrective feedback; vocal emphasis on the conjunction
Child	"Milk and cookies."	A correct response
Clinician	"Very good! You said, *milk **and** cookies*!"	Verbal praise

Repeat the trials until the child gives 5 consecutively correct, imitated responses. When the child imitates 5 correct responses in sequence, fade the modeling. Always point to the target object before asking a question.

Scripts for Fading the Modeling		Note
Clinician	[showing the paired picture of milk and cookies] "What two things do you see? Say, *milk* . . ."	Partial modeling only
Child	"Milk" ["Cookies."]	A wrong response
Clinician	"No, that is not correct. Milk **and** cookies. Don't forget *and* in between. What two things do you see? Say, *Milk* . . ."	Corrective feedback and partial modeling
Child	"Milk and cookies."	A correct response
Clinician	"Very good! You said, *milk **and** cookies*!"	Verbal praise
Clinician	"What two things do you see?"	**An Evoked Trial**
Child	"Milk and cookies."	Correct answer

If the wrong responses persist on 4 to 5 evoked trials, reinstate partial or full modeling for a few trials, again fade the modeling, and re-present the evoked trials.

When the child meets the tentative learning criterion of 10 consecutively correct, nonimitated responses for a given exemplar, move on to the next exemplar. With this procedure, teach 8 to 10 exemplars. Use different exemplars as you see fit for a given child. Use the exemplars and the recording sheet given on the next page (or copy it from the CD).

Conjunction *and* in Phrases

Exemplars and Treatment Recording Sheet

Print this page from the CD or photocopy this page for your clinical use.

Name/Age:	Date:
Goal: Production of the conjunction *and* in phrases with 90% accuracy when asked questions while showing a picture.	Clinician:

Clinician's Comments:

Scoring: Correct: ✓   Incorrect or no response: X

Target skills	Discrete Trials														
	1	2	3	4	5	6	7	8	9	10	11	12	13	14	15
1. milk and cookies															
2. a lion and a tiger															
3. paper and pencil															
4. man and woman															
5. table and chair															
6. spoons and forks															
7. cars and trucks															
8. boys and girls															
9. worms and ants															
10. pie and pizza															

Teach 8 to 10 exemplars each to a training criterion of 10 consecutively correct, nonimitated responses. Then, shift training to the sentence level. Before teaching the conjunction in sentences, baserate their productions; use the protocols that follow.

Conjunction *and* in Sentences

Baserate Protocols

Scripts for Evoked Baserate Trial		Note
Clinician	[showing the paired picture of milk and cookies] "What two things do you see?"	No modeling
Child	"Cookies." ["Milk."]	Scored as a wrong response
Clinician	Scores the response as incorrect.	No corrective feedback
Clinician	[Showing the paired picture of lions and tigers] "What two animals do you see?"	The next trial
Child	"A lion and a tiger."	A correct response
Clinician	Records the response as correct.	No verbal praise

Administer the modeled baserate trials only after completing the evoked trials on all 20 (or more) exemplars.

Scripts for Modeled Baserate Trial		Note
Clinician	[showing the paired picture of milk and cookies] "What two things do you see?" Say, *I see milk and cookies.*"	Modeling
Child	"I see milk. Cookies"	A wrong response
Clinician	Records the response as incorrect.	No corrective feedback
Clinician	[showing the paired picture of lions and tigers] "What two animals do you see?" Say, *I see a lion and a tiger.*"	Modeling
Child	"I see a lion and a tiger."	A correct response
Clinician	Records the response.	No verbal praise

Baserate at least 20 exemplars as shown on the next page.

Conjunction *and* in Sentences

Exemplars and Baserate Recording Sheet

Print this page from the CD or photocopy this page for your clinical use.

Name/Age:	Date:
Goal: To establish the baserates of conjunction *and* in sentences when asked questions while showing a picture.	Clinician:

Clinician's Comments:

Scoring: Correct: ✓   Incorrect or no response: X

Conjunction *and* in Sentences	Evoked	Modeled
1. I see milk and cookies.		
2. I see a lion and a tiger.		
3. I see paper and pencil.		
4. I see a man and a woman.		
5. I see a table and a chair.		
6. I see spoons and forks.		
7. I see cars and trucks.		
8. I see boys and girls.		
9. I see worms and ants.		
10. I see a pie and a pizza.		
11. I see cups and plates.		
12. I see hats and balloons.		
13. I see bears and lions.		
14. I see shoes and socks.		
15. I see trains and planes.		
16. I see pants and shirts.		
17. I see fruits and vegetables.		
18. I see a baby and a mother.		
19. I see a ball and a bat.		
20. I see a cow and a calf.		
Percent correct baserate		

Replace or add new exemplars as you see fit for a given child.

After establishing the baserates for the target sentences, initiate treatment. Use the protocols given on the next page.

Conjunction *and* in Sentences

Treatment Protocols

Scripts for Modeled Discrete Trial Training		Note
Clinician	[showing the paired picture of milk and cookies] "What two things do you see here?" Say, *I see milk **and** cookies*."	Vocal emphasis on the target conjunction
Child	"I see Milk. Cookies"	Scored as a wrong response
Clinician	"No, you forgot the **and**. What two things do you see? Say, *I see milk **and** cookies*."	Corrective feedback; vocal emphasis on the target conjunction
Child	"I see milk and cookies."	Scored as correct
Clinician	"Very good! You said, *I see milk **and** cookies*!"	Verbal praise

Repeat the trials until the child gives 5 consecutively correct, imitated responses. When the child imitates 5 correct responses in sequence, fade the modeling.

Scripts for Fading the Modeling		Note
Clinician	[showing the paired picture of milk and cookies] "What two things do you see here? Say, *I see . . .*"	Partial modeling only
Child	"Cookies. Milk"	A wrong response
Clinician	"No, you forgot the whole sentence and you didn't say *and*. What two things do you see? Say, *I see cookies . . .*"	Corrective feedback and partial modeling
Child	"I see milk and cookies."	A correct response
Clinician	"Very good! You said, *I see milk **and** cookies*!"	Verbal praise
Clinician	"What two things do you see?"	**An Evoked Trial**
Child	"I see milk and cookies."	Correct answer
Clinician	"Excellent! You said the whole sentence!"	Verbal praise

Conjunction *and* in Sentences

Exemplars and Treatment Recording Sheet

Print this page from the CD or photocopy this page for your clinical use.

Name/Age:	Date:
Goal: Production of the conjunction *and* in sentences with 90% accuracy when asked questions while showing a picture.	Clinician:

Clinician's Comments:

Scoring: Correct: ✓   Incorrect or no response: X

Target skills	Discrete Trials														
	1	2	3	4	5	6	7	8	9	10	11	12	13	14	15
1. I see milk and cookies.															
2. I see lions and tigers.															
3. I see paper and pencil.															
4. I see a man and a woman.															
5. I see a table and a chair.															
6. I see spoons and forks.															
7. I see cars and trucks.															
8. I see boys and girls.															
9. I see worms and ants.															
10. I see a pie and a pizza.															

When the child has met the learning criterion of 10 consecutively correct, evoked (nonimitated) responses for each of the 10 target sentences, conduct a probe to see if the production of the conjunction has generalized to untrained stimuli. Use the probe protocols given on the next page (or print it from the CD).

Conjunction *and* in Sentences

Probe Protocols and Recording Sheet

Print this page from the CD or photocopy this page for your clinical use.

On the probes, present the untrained exemplars (UT). When the child fails to meet the 90% correct probe criterion, either teach 2 to 4 new exemplars or give additional training trials on already trained exemplars. If needed, select new exemplars for probes. Probe at least 10 untrained exemplars. Alternate probes and treatment until the probe criterion is met.

Scripts for Probe Trials

Clinician	[Presents a paired untrained stimulus: cups and plates] "What two things do you see here? Start with *I see . . .*"	No modeling; only a prompt
Child	"I see cups and plates."	A correct, generalized response
Clinician	Scores the response as correct.	Offers no reinforcement
Clinician	[Presents another untrained stimulus pair hats and balloons] "What two things do you see here? Start with *I see . . .*"	The second probe trial
Child	"Hats. Balloons."	A wrong probe response
Clinician	Scores the response as incorrect.	Offers no corrective feedback

Name:	Date:	Session #:
Age:	**Clinician:**	
Disorder: Language	**Target: Conjunction *and* in sentences (Probe)**	
Untrained Stimuli	**Score: + correct; – incorrect or no responses**	
1. I see cups and plates. (UT)		
2. I see hats and balloons. (UT)		
3. I see bears and lions. (UT)		
4. I see shoes and socks. (UT)		
5. I see trains and planes.(UT)		
6. I see pants and shirts. (UT)		
7. I see fruits and vegetables. (UT)		
8. I see a baby and a mother. (UT)		
9. I see a ball and a bat. (UT)		
10. I see a cow and a calf. (UT)		
Percent correct probe (Criterion: 90%)		

If the child does not meet the probe criterion, give additional training on the trained sentences, or teach new exemplars. Subsequently, readminister the probe trials. When the child meets 90% correct probe criterion, teach another morphologic feature or shift training to conversational speech in which the production of the conjunction is monitored and reinforced.

Conjunction *because*
Conjunction *because* in Sentences
Baserating Protocols

Scripts for Evoked Baserate Trial		Note
Clinician	[showing the picture of a boy eating pizza] "He is eating pizza because he is hungry. Why is he eating pizza? Start with *he is eating pizza because* . . ."	Prompting directs the child toward the target skill
Child	"He likes it." ["He is hungry."]	Scored as a wrong response
Clinician	Scores the response as incorrect.	No corrective feedback
Clinician	[Showing the picture of a girl drinking water] "She is drinking water because she is thirsty. Why is she drinking water? Start with *she is drinking water because* . . ."	The next trial
Child	"She is drinking water because she is thirsty."	A correct response
Clinician	Records the response as correct.	No verbal praise

Administer the modeled baserate trials only after completing the evoked trials on all 20 (or more) exemplars.

Scripts for Modeled Baserate Trial		Note
Clinician	[showing the picture of a boy eating pizza] "He is eating pizza. Why is he eating pizza? Say, *he is eating pizza because he is hungry.*"	Modeling
Child	"He is hungry." ["He is eating."]	A wrong response
Clinician	Records the response as incorrect.	No corrective feedback
Clinician	[Showing the picture of a girl drinking water] "She is drinking. Why is she drinking water? Say, *she is drinking water because she is thirsty.*"	Modeling
Child	"She is drinking water because she is thirsty."	A correct response
Clinician	Records the response.	No verbal praise

Baserate at least 20 exemplars as shown on the next page.

Conjunction *because* in Sentences

Exemplars and Baserate Recording Sheet

Print this page from the CD or photocopy this page for your clinical use.

Name/Age:	Date:
Goal: To establish the baserates of conjunction *because* in sentences when asked questions while showing a picture.	Clinician:

Clinician's Comments:

Scoring: Correct: ✓   Incorrect or no response: X

Conjunction *because* in Sentences	Evoked	Modeled
1. He is eating pizza because he is hungry.		
2. She is drinking water because she is thirsty.		
3. He is wearing a jacket because it is cold.		
4. She is wearing sunglasses because it is sunny.		
5. He is yawning because he is tired.		
6. She is washing her car because it is dirty.		
7. He is packing because he is going somewhere.		
8. She is sleeping because it is night.		
9. He is buying candy because he likes it.		
10. She is sad because her toy is broke.		
11. He is running because the policeman is chasing.		
12. She is happy because she got a gift.		
13. He is spraying water because the house is on fire.		
14. She is scratching because she is itching.		
15. He is smiling because he is happy.		
16. She is searching because he lost his puppy.		
17. He is wiping the table because it is dirty.		
18. She is swimming because she is hot.		
19. He is shouting because they can't hear him.		
20. She is laughing because he told a joke.		
Percent correct baserate		

Replace or add new exemplars as you see fit for a given child.

After establishing the baserates for the target sentences, initiate treatment. Use the protocols given on the next page.

Conjunction *because* in Sentences

Treatment Protocols

Scripts for Modeled Discrete Trial Training		Note
Clinician	[showing the picture of a boy eating pizza] "He is eating pizza. Why is he eating pizza? Say, *he is eating pizza **because** he is hungry*."	Vocal emphasis on the target word
Child	"He is hungry." ["He is eating."]	Scored as a wrong response
Clinician	"No, you didn't say the whole sentence. Remember ***because***. Why is he eating pizza? Say, *he is eating pizza **because** he is hungry*."	Corrective feedback; vocal emphasis on the target word
Child	"He is eating pizza because he is hungry."	Scored as correct
Clinician	"Very good! You said the whole sentence! You didn't forget ***because***!"	Verbal praise

Repeat the trials until the child gives 5 consecutively correct, imitated responses. When the child imitates 5 correct responses in sequence, fade the modeling.

Scripts for Fading the Modeling		Note
Clinician	[showing the picture of a boy eating pizza] "He is eating pizza. Why is he eating pizza? Say, *he is eating pizza . . .*"	Partial modeling only
Child	"He is eating pizza." ["He is hungry."]	A wrong response
Clinician	"No, you forgot the whole sentence and you didn't say *because*. Why is he eating pizza? Say, *he is eating pizza . . .*"	Corrective feedback and partial modeling
Child	"He is eating pizza because he is hungry."	A correct response
Clinician	"Very good! You said the whole sentence! You didn't forget ***because***!"	Verbal praise
Clinician	"Why is he eating pizza?"	**An Evoked Trial**
Child	"He is eating pizza because he is hungry."	Correct answer
Clinician	"Excellent! You said the whole sentence!"	Verbal praise

Conjunction *because* in Sentences

Exemplars and Treatment Recording Sheet

Print this page from the CD or photocopy this page for your clinical use.

Name/Age:	Date:
Goal: Production of the conjunction *because* in sentences with 90% accuracy when asked questions while showing a picture.	Clinician:

Clinician's Comments:

Scoring: Correct: ✓   Incorrect or no response: X

Target skills	Discrete Trials														
	1	2	3	4	5	6	7	8	9	10	11	12	13	14	15
1. He is eating pizza because he is hungry.															
2. She is drinking water because she is thirsty.															
3. He is wearing a jacket because it is cold.															
4. She is wearing sunglasses because it is sunny.															
5. He is yawning because he is tired.															
6. She is washing her car because it is dirty.															
7. He is packing because he is going somewhere.															
8. She is sleeping because it is night.															
9. He is buying candy because he likes it.															
10. She is sad because her toy is broken.															

When the child has met the learning criterion of 10 consecutively correct, evoked (nonimitated) responses for each of the 10 target sentences, conduct a probe to see if the production of the conjunction has generalized to untrained stimuli. Use the probe protocol given on the next page (or print it from the CD).

Conjunction *because* in Sentences
Probe Protocols and Recording Sheet

Print this page from the CD or photocopy this page for your clinical use.

On the probes, present the untrained exemplars (UT). When the child fails to meet the 90% correct probe criterion, either teach 2 to 4 new exemplars or give additional training trials on already trained exemplars. If needed, select new exemplars for probes. Probe at least 10 untrained exemplars. Alternate probes and treatment until the probe criterion is met.

Scripts for Probe Trials

Clinician	[Presents an untrained stimulus: a man running, a policeman chasing] "Why is this man running? Start with, *the man is running because . . .*"	No modeling; only a prompt
Child	"The man is running because the policeman is chasing."	A correct, generalized response
Clinician	Scores the response as correct.	Offers no reinforcement
Clinician	[presents the picture of a happy girl receiving a packaged gift] "Why is she happy? Start with *she is happy because . . .*"	The second probe trial
Child	"She got a gift." [She is happy because.]	A wrong probe response
Clinician	Scores the response as incorrect.	Offers no corrective feedback

Name:	Date:	Session #:	
Age:	Clinician:		
Disorder: Language	Target: Conjunction *because* in sentences (Probe)		
Untrained Stimuli		Score: + correct; − incorrect or no responses	
1. He is running because the policeman is chasing. (UT)			
2. She is happy because she got a gift. (UT)			
3. He is spraying water because the house is on fire. (UT)			
4. She is scratching because she is itching. (UT)			
5. He is smiling because he is happy. (UT)			
6. She is searching because she lost her puppy. (UT)			
7. He is wiping the table because it is dirty. (UT)			
8. She is swimming because she is hot. (UT)			
9. He is shouting because they can't hear him. (UT)			
10. She is laughing because he told her a joke. (UT)			
Percent correct probe (Criterion: 90%)			

If the child does not meet the probe criterion, give additional training on the trained sentences, or teach new exemplars. Subsequently, readminister the probe trials. When the child meets 90% correct probe criterion, teach another morphologic feature or shift training to conversational speech in which the production of the conjunction is monitored and reinforced.

Conjunction *but*
Conjunction *but* in Basic Sentences
Baserate Protocols

Scripts for Evoked Baserate Trial		Note
Clinician	[showing the picture of a boy getting a glass of juice] "He asked for milk, but his mom gave him juice. What happened? Start with *he asked for milk, but . . .*"	Prompting directs the child toward the target skill
Child	"He got juice." ["Asked for milk, got juice."]	Scored as a wrong response
Clinician	Scores the response as incorrect.	No corrective feedback
Clinician	[showing the picture of a girl pushing chocolate away from her] "This girl has a problem. She likes chocolate, but she can't eat it. What is her problem? Start with *she likes chocolate, but . . .*"	The next trial
Child	"She likes chocolate, but can't eat it."	A correct response
Clinician	Records the response as correct.	No verbal praise

Administer the modeled baserate trials only after completing the evoked trials on all 20 (or more) exemplars.

Scripts for Modeled Baserate Trial		Note
Clinician	[showing the picture of a boy getting a glass of juice] "He asked for milk, but his mom gave him juice. What happened? Say, *he asked for milk, but he got juice.*"	Modeling
Child	"He got juice."	A wrong response
Clinician	Records the response as incorrect.	No corrective feedback
Clinician	[showing the picture of a girl pushing chocolate away from her] "This girl has a problem. She likes chocolate, but she can't eat it. What is her problem? Say, *she likes chocolate, but can't eat it.*"	Modeling
Child	"She likes chocolate, but can't eat it."	A correct response
Clinician	Records the response.	No verbal praise

Baserate at least 20 exemplars as shown on the next page.

Conjunction *but* in Basic Sentences

Exemplars and Baserate Recording Sheet

Print this page from the CD or photocopy this page for your clinical use.

Name/Age:	Date:
Goal: To establish the baserates of conjunction *but* in basic sentences when asked questions while showing a picture.	Clinician:

Clinician's Comments:

Scoring: Correct: ✓   Incorrect or no response: X

Conjunction *but* in Sentences	Evoked	Modeled
1. He asked for milk, but got juice.		
2. She likes chocolate, but can't eat it.		
3. He wanted to go to the circus, but didn't.		
4. She went to the zoo, but didn't see lions.		
5. The boy was sick, but went to school.		
6. The woman went fishing, but did not catch fish.		
7. The girl wanted the toy, but she didn't buy it.		
8. He turned on the radio, but it was broken.		
9. She likes her coat, but it is short.		
10. The boy likes the cake, but didn't eat it.		
11. He wanted to swim, but didn't.		
12. She wanted to paint, but she has no paper.		
13. She wants to play, but she can't.		
14. He wants the balloon, but he can't get it.		
15. She wanted to dance, but there was no music.		
16. The girl went to the party, but she was bored because there were no kids.		
17. The boy was dry, but his bag was wet.		
18. He wanted to go home, but he couldn't.		
19. She wants to buy candy, but has no money.		
20. He went to class, but no one was there.		
Percent correct baserate		

After establishing the baserates for the target sentences, initiate treatment. Use the protocols given on the next page.

Conjunction *but* in Basic Sentences

Treatment Protocols

Scripts for Modeled Discrete Trial Training		Note
Clinician	[showing the picture of a boy getting a glass of juice] "He asked for milk, but his mom gave him juice. What happened? Say, *he asked for milk,* **but** *he got juice.*"	Vocal emphasis on the target word
Child	"He got juice." ["Mom gave him juice."]	Scored as a wrong response
Clinician	"No, you didn't say the whole sentence. Remember **but**. What happened? Say, *he asked for milk,* **but** *got juice.*"	Corrective feedback; vocal emphasis on the target word
Child	"He asked for milk, but got juice."	Scored as correct
Clinician	"Very good! You said the whole sentence! You didn't forget **but**!"	Verbal praise

Repeat the trials until the child gives 5 consecutively correct, imitated responses. When the child imitates 5 correct responses in sequence, fade the modeling.

Scripts for Fading the Modeling		Note
Clinician	[showing the picture of a boy getting a glass of juice] "He asked for milk, but his mom gave him juice. What happened? Say, *he asked for milk, . . .*"	Partial modeling only
Child	"He got juice."	A wrong response
Clinician	"No, you forgot the whole sentence and you didn't say but. What happened? Say, *he asked for milk, . . .*"	Corrective feedback and partial modeling
Child	"He asked for milk, but he got juice."	A correct response
Clinician	"Very good! You said the whole sentence! You didn't forget **but**!"	Verbal praise
Clinician	"What happened?"	**An Evoked Trial**
Child	"He asked for milk, but got juice."	Correct answer
Clinician	"Excellent! You said the whole sentence!"	Verbal praise

Conjunction *but* in Basic Sentences

Exemplars and Treatment Recording Sheet

Print this page from the CD or photocopy this page for your clinical use.

Name/Age:	Date:
Goal: Production of the conjunction *but* in basic sentences with 90% accuracy when asked questions while showing a picture.	Clinician:

Clinician's Comments:

Scoring: Correct: ✓   Incorrect or no response: X

Target skills	Discrete Trials														
	1	2	3	4	5	6	7	8	9	10	11	12	13	14	15
1. He asked for milk, but got juice.															
2. She likes chocolate, but can't eat it.															
3. He wanted to go to the circus, but didn't.															
4. She went to the zoo, but didn't see lions.															
5. The boy was sick, but went to school.															
6. The woman went fishing, but did not catch fish.															
7. The girl wanted the toy, but she didn't buy it.															
8. He turned on the radio, but it was broken.															
9. She likes her coat, but it is short.															
10. The boy likes the cake, but didn't eat it.															

When the child has met the learning criterion of 10 consecutively correct, evoked (nonimitated) responses for each of the 10 target sentences, conduct a probe to see if the production of the conjunction has generalized to untrained stimuli. Use the probe protocols given on the next page (or print it from the CD).

Conjunction *but* in Basic Sentences
Probe Protocols and Recording Sheet

Print this page from the CD or photocopy this page for your clinical use.

On the probes, present the untrained exemplars (UT). When the child fails to meet the 90% correct probe criterion, either teach 2 to 4 new exemplars or give additional training trials on already trained exemplars. If needed, select new exemplars for probes. Probe at least 10 untrained exemplars. Alternate probes and treatment until the probe criterion is met.

Scripts for Probe Trials

Clinician	[Presents an untrained stimulus: a man in swim trunks standing near a pool] "He wanted to swim, but didn't. What is this man's problem? Start with, *he wanted to swim . . .*"	No modeling; only a prompt
Child	"He wanted to swim, but didn't."	A correct, generalized response
Clinician	Scores the response as correct.	Offers no reinforcement
Clinician	[presents the picture of a girl with paint and paint brush, but with no paper on the easel] "She wanted to paint, but she has no paper. What is her problem? Start with *she wanted to paint . . .*"	The second probe trial
Child	"She has no paper." ["No paper."]	A wrong probe response
Clinician	Scores the response as incorrect.	Offers no corrective feedback

Name:	Date:	Session #:
Age:	**Clinician:**	
Disorder: Language	**Target: Conjunction *but* in basic sentences (Probe)**	

Untrained Stimuli	Score: + correct; – incorrect or no responses
1. He wanted to swim, but didn't. (UT)	
2. She wanted to paint, but she has no paper. (UT)	
3. She wants to play, but she can't. (UT)	
4. He wants the balloon, but he can't get it. (UT)	
5. She wanted to dance, but there was no music. (UT)	
6. The girl went to the party, but she was bored because there were no kids. (UT)	
7. The boy was dry, but his bag was wet. (UT)	
8. He wanted to go home, but he couldn't. (UT)	
9. She wants to buy candy, but has no money. (UT)	
10. He went to class, but no one was there. (UT)	
Percent correct probe (Criterion: 90%)	

If the child does not meet the probe criterion, give additional training on the trained sentences, or teach new exemplars. Subsequently, readminister the probe trials. When the child meets 90% correct probe criterion, teach another morphologic feature or shift training to conversational speech in which the production of the conjunction is monitored and reinforced.

Conjunction *but* in Expanded Sentences

Baserate Protocols

Scripts for Evoked Baserate Trial		Note
Clinician	[showing the picture of a boy getting a glass of juice] "He asked for milk, but his mom gave him juice because there was no milk. What happened? Start with *he asked for milk, but got juice because . . .*"	Prompting directs the child toward the target skill
Child	"He got juice." ["Asked for milk, got juice."]	Scored as a wrong response
Clinician	Scores the response as incorrect.	No corrective feedback
Clinician	[showing the picture of a girl pushing a piece of chocolate away from her] "This girl has a problem. She likes chocolate, but she can't eat it because her Mom says 'no.' What is her problem? Start with *she likes chocolate, but can't eat it because . . .*"	The next trial
Child	"She likes chocolate, but can't eat it because her Mom says 'no.'"	A correct response
Clinician	Records the response as correct.	No verbal praise

Administer the modeled baserate trials only after completing the evoked trials on all 20 (or more) exemplars.

Scripts for Modeled Baserate Trial		Note
Clinician	[showing the picture of a boy getting a glass of juice] "He asked for milk, but his mom gave him juice because there was no milk. What happened? Say, *he asked for milk, but he got juice because there was no milk.*"	Modeling
Child	"He asked for milk, but got juice."	A wrong response
Clinician	Records the response as incorrect.	No corrective feedback
Clinician	[showing the picture of a girl pushing a piece of chocolate away from her] "This girl ha a problem. She likes chocolate, but she can't eat it because her Mom says 'no.' What is her problem? Say, *she likes chocolate, but can't eat it because her Mom says 'no.'*"	Modeling
Child	"She likes chocolate, but can't eat it because her Mom says 'no'."	A correct response
Clinician	Records the response.	No verbal praise

Baserate at least 20 exemplars as shown on the next page.

Conjunction *but* in Expanded Sentences

Exemplars and Baserate Recording Sheet

Print this page from the CD or photocopy this page for your clinical use.

Name/Age:	Date:
Goal: To establish the baserates of conjunction *but* in expanded sentences when asked questions while showing a picture.	Clinician:

Clinician's Comments:

Scoring: Correct: ✓   Incorrect or no response: X

Conjunction *but* in Sentences	Evoked	Modeled
1. He asked for milk, but got juice because there was no milk.		
2. She likes chocolate, but can't eat it because her mother says "no."		
3. He wanted to go to the circus, but didn't because his dad had no time.		
4. She went to the zoo, but didn't see lions because they were hiding.		
5. The boy was sick, but went to school because he likes school.		
6. The woman went fishing, but did not catch fish because she didn't have worms.		
7. The girl wanted the toy, but she didn't buy it because it cost too much.		
8. He turned on the radio, but it was broken because he had dropped it.		
9. She likes her coat, but it is short because she grew taller.		
10. The boy likes the cake, but didn't eat it because it is too sweet.		
11. He wanted to swim, but didn't because it is cold.		
12. She wanted to paint, but she has no paper because she didn't buy it.		
13. She wants to play, but she can't because she has homework to do.		
14. He wants the balloon, but he can't get it because it is too high.		
15. She wanted to dance, but there was no music because the radio was broken.		
16. The girl went to the party, but she was bored because there were no kids.		
17. The boy was dry, but his bag was wet because he did not cover it.		
18. He wanted to go home, but he couldn't because he did not have the key.		
19. She wants to buy candy, but has no money because she spent it.		
20. He went to class, but no one was there because it was a holiday.		
Percent correct baserate		

After establishing the baserates for the target sentences, initiate treatment. Use the protocols given on the next page.

Conjunction *but* in Expanded Sentences

Treatment Protocols

Scripts for Modeled Discrete Trial Training		Note
Clinician	[showing the picture of a boy getting a glass of juice] "He asked for milk, but his mom gave him juice because there was no milk. What happened? Say, *he asked for milk, **but** he got juice because there was no milk.*"	Vocal emphasis on the target word
Child	"He asked for milk, but got juice." ["Mom gave him juice."]	Scored as a wrong response
Clinician	"No, you didn't say the whole sentence. Remember, **but**. What happened? Say, *he asked for milk, **but** got juice, because there was no milk.*"	Corrective feedback; vocal emphasis on the target word
Child	"He asked for milk, but got juice because there was no milk."	Scored as correct
Clinician	"Very good! You said the whole sentence! You didn't forget, **but**!"	Verbal praise

Repeat the trials until the child gives 5 consecutively correct, imitated responses. When the child imitates 5 correct responses in sequence, fade the modeling.

Scripts for Fading the Modeling		Note
Clinician	[showing the picture of a boy getting a glass of juice] "He asked for milk, but his mom gave him juice because there was no milk. What happened? Say, *he asked for milk, but he got juice because. . .*"	Partial modeling only
Child	"He asked for milk but he got juice."	A wrong response
Clinician	"No, you forgot the whole sentence. What happened? Say, *he asked for milk, but got juice because . . .*"	Corrective feedback and partial modeling
Child	"He asked for milk, but got juice because there was no milk."	A correct response
Clinician	"Very good! You said the whole sentence! You didn't forget, **but**!"	Verbal praise
Clinician	"What did the boy ask and why did the Mom give him juice?"	**An Evoked Trial**
Child	"He asked for milk, but got juice because there was no milk."	Correct answer
Clinician	"Excellent! You said the whole sentence!"	Verbal praise

Conjunction *but* in Expanded Sentences
Exemplars and Treatment Recording Sheet

Print this page from the CD or photocopy this page for your clinical use.

Name/Age:	Date:
Goal: Production of the conjunction *but* in expanded sentences with 90% accuracy when asked questions while showing a picture.	Clinician:

Clinician's Comments:

Scoring: Correct: ✓   Incorrect or no response: X

Target skills	Discrete Trials														
	1	2	3	4	5	6	7	8	9	10	11	12	13	14	15
1. He asked for milk, but got juice because there was no milk.															
2. She likes chocolate, but can't eat it because her mother says "no."															
3. He wanted to go to the circus, but didn't because his dad had no time.															
4. She went to the zoo, but didn't see lions because they were hiding.															
5. The boy was sick, but went to school because he likes school.															
6. The woman went fishing, but did not catch fish because she didn't have worms.															
7. The girl wanted the toy, but she didn't buy it because it cost too much.															
8. He turned on the radio, but it was broken because he had dropped it.															
9. She likes her coat, but it is short because she grew taller.															
10. The boy likes the cake, but didn't eat it because it is too sweet.															

When the child has met the learning criterion of 10 consecutively correct, evoked (nonimitated) responses for each of the 10 target sentences, conduct a probe to see if the production of the conjunction has generalized to untrained stimuli. Use the protocols given on the next page (or print it from the CD).

Conjunction *but* in Expanded Sentences
Probe Protocols and Recording Sheet

Print this page from the CD or photocopy this page for your clinical use.

On the probes, present the untrained exemplars (UT). When the child fails to meet the 90% correct probe criterion, either teach 2 to 4 new exemplars or give additional training trials on already trained exemplars. If needed, select new exemplars for probes. Probe at least 10 untrained exemplars. Alternate probes and treatment until the probe criterion is met.

Scripts for Probe Trials

Clinician	[Presents an untrained stimulus: a man in swim trunks standing near a pool] "He wanted to swim, but didn't because it is cold. What is this man's problem? Start with, *he wanted to swim . . .*"	No modeling; only a prompt
Child	"He wanted to swim, but didn't."	A correct, generalized response
Clinician	Scores the response as correct.	Offers no reinforcement
Clinician	[presents the picture of a girl with paint and paint brush, but with no paper on the easel] "She wanted to paint, but didn't because she has no paper. What is her problem? Start with *she wants to paint . . .*"	The second probe trial
Child	"She has no paper." ["No paper."]	A wrong probe response
Clinician	Scores the response as incorrect.	Offers no corrective feedback

Name:	**Date:**	**Session #:**
Age:	**Clinician:**	
Disorder: Language	**Target: Conjunction *but* in expanded sentences (Probe)**	
Untrained Stimuli	**Score: + correct; – incorrect or no responses**	
1. He wanted to swim, but didn't because it is cold. (UT)		
2. She wanted to paint, but didn't because she has no paper. (UT)		
3. She wants to play, but she can't because she has homework to do. (UT)		
4. He wants the balloon, but he can't get it because it is too high. (UT)		
5. She wanted to dance, but there was no music because the radio was broken. (UT)		
6. The girl went to the party, but she was bored because there were no kids. (UT)		
7. The boy was dry, but his bag was wet because he did not cover it. (UT)		
8. He wanted to go home, but he couldn't because he did not have the key. (UT)		
9. She wants to buy candy, but has no money because she spent it. (UT)		
10. He went to class, but no one was there because it was a holiday. (UT)		
Percent correct probe (Criterion: 90%)		

If the child does not meet the probe criterion, give additional training on the trained sentences, or teach new exemplars. Subsequently, readminister the probe trials. When the child meets 90% correct probe criterion, teach another morphologic feature or shift training to conversational speech in which the production of the conjunction is monitored and reinforced.

Glossary

Autism: A form of pervasive developmental disorder that may be mild to very severe; marked by disinterest in typical social interaction, severely impaired communication skills, and stereotypical movements; also known as autism spectrum disorder (ASD); language disorders are common, and behavioral treatment is known to be the most effective of the alternatives.

Baseline or **baserates:** A measure of target skills established before treatment is begun; no reinforcement or corrective feedback is offered during baseline trials; helps document improvement in skills in treatment sessions.

Behavioral treatment: An efficient method of treating language skills in which the clinician manages an interdependent relationship between antecedent events (stimuli that include instructions, pictures, modeling, and prompting), specified language skills, and consequences in the form of listener reactions; consequences are often verbal praise and corrective feedback, but may also include tokens, free time, and food items.

Booster treatment: Treatment offered any time after an initial dismissal; necessary to maintain language skills; booster treatment is usually brief.

Bound morphemes: Suffixes and prefixes that are attached to a root word (e.g., the regular plural *s* or the present progressive *ing*); do not convey much meaning when they stand alone.

Child-specific (client-specific) measurement: Measurement of a client's specific behaviors under conditions that are relevant to the child and his or her cultural and family background.

Cloze: Also known as the sentence completion method in which the clinician starts a sentence and pauses to give the child a chance to complete it; the same as **partial model;** useful in fading a full model of the target behavior.

Communication: Traditionally defined as exchange of information between two or more persons in verbal, gestural, written, and other forms; verbal or nonverbal behavior; often, talking, gesturing, using sign language, or using technical means to interact socially (as in the use of a communication board).

Conditioned generalized reinforcement: Use of reinforcers whose effects are due to past learning and are independent of a particular state of motivation (desire); the use of a token system; because the tokens may be exchanged for a variety of objects the child may desire, the child is always motivated in a token system.

Conditioned generalized reinforcers: Tokens and such other consequences that may be exchanged for a wide variety of reinforcers; known to be effective in treating communication disorders, including language disorders.

Connotative meaning: Emotional meanings the words suggest but do not directly state.

Contingency priming: Also known as **reinforcement recruitment;** teaching a child or an adult client to seek attention to his or her newly learned desirable behaviors from people who fail to reinforce; known to be effective in helping clients maintain skills in natural settings.

Continuous schedule of reinforcement: A method of reinforcement delivery in which all correct responses are reinforced; effective in establishing the target behavior; needs to be faded in later stages of reinforcement to promote maintenance of target skills that are not reinforced continuously in the natural environment.

Controlled conversation: Conversation in which the clinician takes a more direct role than usual to establish certain skills; eventually, to be faded into more naturalistic conversation in which the child speaks spontaneously.

Controlled research: A type of research (including treatment research) in which treatment is compared against no treatment and may involve either a group experimental design or a single-subject experimental design; necessary to establish the efficacy of a treatment procedure.

Conversational repair: A pragmatic language skill necessary to restore meaningful communication when communication breakdowns occur; includes such skills as asking for clarification and restating a message in different words when listeners fail to understand.

Conversational turn taking: A pragmatic language skill in which the conversational partners take the role of listeners and talkers in a socially acceptable manner.

Corrective feedback: Letting the child know that a response he or she just made was wrong, inappropriate, inefficient, and so forth; necessary to decrease incorrect or inappropriate behaviors during treatment.

Delay: Setting up communicative situations and then waiting for the child to respond in the expectation that the child will spontaneously respond; a technique used in the milieu approach to teach a child to respond to environmental stimuli other than listener attention as cues for verbalization.

Delayed assistance: Delaying assistance to a child who needs it in the expectation that the child will speak or act without the clinician's assistance; helps promote spontaneity of communication.

Differential reinforcement: A procedure to teach discriminated responses (e.g., the response "red" to a *red stimulus* and "green" to a *green stimulus* or "cup" to a singular item and "cups" to plural items); essential in teaching language concepts.

Differential Reinforcement of Alternative Behavior (DRA): Teaching a desirable behavior that accesses the same reinforcer as an undesirable behavior; for instance, if the child gets food or toys by whining or pointing (not making requests), the clinician may give the desired item only when the child makes a request; an alternative, desirable behavior replaces the undesirable behavior.

Differential Reinforcement of Incompatible Behavior (DRI): Reinforcing a desirable behavior that is incompatible with a frequently exhibited undesirable behavior; for instance, if a boy tends to leave his chair during treatment, he may be praised or given a token just for sitting, which is incompatible with leaving the chair; known to be effective in reducing undesirable behaviors during treatment sessions.

Differential Reinforcement of Low Rates (DRL): Reinforcing a child for reducing the frequency of an undesirable behavior; for instance, a child may be reinforced for asking "are we done yet?" only once in a 20-minute duration as against once every 5 minutes (baserate).

Differential Reinforcement of Other Behavior (DRO): Reinforcing one of several desirable behaviors to reduce a particular undesirable behavior; for instance, a boy who leaves his chair during treatment may be reinforced for sitting quietly, looking at the pictures or other stimuli, listening to a story, or coloring a book; the boy will be told that he will not receive the reinforcement if he leaves his chair; only the behavior to be reduced is specified; those that will be reinforced are many and are often unspecified; known to be effective in reducing undesirable behaviors.

Direct replication: A type of treatment research in which the same researcher repeats his or her own earlier study with little or no modification in the treatment procedure to see if the results are reliable; most of the behavioral treatment techniques described in the protocols have been directly replicated and shown to produce reliable results.

Discourse: Conversation, storytelling, and such other complex verbal interactions between two or more individuals; often described as pragmatic language skill; treatment target for most older students and younger children who have mastered the basic morphologic features and general sentence structures.

Discrete trials: A highly researched behavioral treatment procedure in which the client is given repeated and temporally separated opportunities to produce a response; often a discrete trial includes instructions, exhibition of pictures or other stimuli, questions, modeling, and prompts that the clinician delivers and then waits for a few seconds for the child to respond; each attempt the child makes is scored as correct or wrong; trials are repeated until the child meets a learning criterion; known to be efficient and effective in establishing various skills, including language skills in children (and adults); helps measure skills reliably.

Discriminative stimuli: Stimuli that help evoke a correct response that gets reinforced; most treatment stimuli (including the clinician and the clinical setting) are discriminative stimuli; responses are more likely in their presence than in their absence; including stimuli from home and asking parents to participate in treatment sessions will expand the realm of discriminative stimuli and thus promote generalized productions of language skills.

Echolalia: A parrotlike repetition of what is just heard or has been heard in the past; a common feature of children with autism; a behavior that needs to be reduced or eliminated.

Evidence-based practice: The use of treatment methods that are supported by controlled and replicated research evidence; may include other considerations such as the clinician's best judgment, cost, and social acceptability of the procedures offered.

Evoked trials: Baserate or treatment trials in which the clinician asks a typical question but does not model the correct response; more naturalistic than the imitative trials; when a child gives 10 consecutively correct, evoked responses, the clinician may consider that particular exemplar learned and move on to the next exemplar.

Expressive language: Language production, often contrasted with language comprehension.

Extinction: Terminating the reinforcer for a response while no other attempt is made to stop it; the same as ignoring; is a good choice to reduce such troublesome behaviors as crying in the treatment room or frequent questions the child asks to interrupt treatment (e.g., "Are we done yet?").

Eye contact: Maintenance of mutual eye gaze during conversation; a pragmatic language skill; culturally determined as eye contact during conversation is not expected in all cultures, especially when the conversational partners are an adult and a child; an optional target for children whose family does not insist on eye contact.

Fading: A technique in which such special stimuli as modeling and prompting are gradually withdrawn so that the child can more readily respond spontaneously; treatment protocols include fading of modeling and prompts as the treatment sequence begins with modeling and fades into evoked trials.

Fictional narratives: Telling a story, a well-known fairy tale, or the plot of a popular movie or television show; a pragmatic language skill; appropriate clinical target for older students and younger students who have mastered the essential morphologic features and basic sentence structures.

Figurative meaning: Metaphoric meaning in language; words that normally represent something are used to represent something else (e.g., the saying, *a mountain of trouble*); part of abstract language; appropriate clinical target for older students and younger students who have mastered the essential morphologic features and basic sentence structures.

Final conversational probes: An assessment of generalized production of clinically established target behaviors produced in conversational speech in the clinic and in natural environments; often conducted before dismissing a client from services.

Fixed interval (FI) schedule: A pattern of reinforcement in which a fixed amount of time should elapse before the child is given an opportunity to earn a reinforcer; for instance, in a FI5 schedule, reinforcers are given only when correct responses are separated by 5 seconds or minutes (always specified); not frequently used in teaching language skills.

Fixed ratio (FR) schedule: Frequently used in teaching language skills, an FR schedule is a pattern of reinforcement in which a specific number of responses are required to earn reinforcers; in an FR1 schedule, clinicians reinforce every correct response; in an FR5 schedule, clinicians reinforce every fifth correct response; stretching the ratio gradually is a method of fading explicit reinforcement and helps promote maintenance of clinically established skills.

Follow-up assessment: Any assessment of a client's communication skills following initial dismissal from treatment; necessary to assess response maintenance; when the follow-up assessment shows a decline in target skills, booster therapy may be arranged.

Free morphemes: A morpheme that conveys meaning standing alone and cannot be broken down into smaller parts; most individual words (without prefixes and suffixes) are free morphemes; contrasted with *bound morphemes*.

Functional response classes: Skills that are independent of each other; teaching a few responses belonging to the same class is sufficient to promote generalized production of other responses within the class; responses that belong to different classes need separate training; in language, linguistic categories do not necessarily form response classes; for instance, auxiliary and copula are linguistically separate but they belong to the same response class; teaching either auxiliary or copula is sufficient to generate both; on the other hand, irregular plural is a single linguistic category, but each irregular plural word is a response class unto itself; each word needs to be taught; response classes are clinically more useful concepts than are linguistic categories.

Function words: A category of words that includes such grammatic morphemes as articles, prepositions, and conjunctions; often missing in the language of children with language disorders; useful clinical targets; contrasted with *content words*.

Generalization: A behavioral process in which newly learned responses are extended to new stimuli, new situations, and new linguistic contexts; a desirable clinical goal; probes described in the protocols help assess whether a child who has mastered a language element can now produce it in new contexts (including new stimuli and situations).

Generalized productions: Responses that are given to stimuli not used in training; assessed by probes.

High probability behavior: A behavior that is produced more often and has the power to increase another behavior that is produced less often (as are most language skills in children with language disorders); if access to a high probability behavior (e.g., a child's tendency to play with a new toy) is given only if the child performs a low probability behavior first (e.g., only after the child has worked on language skills for 5 minutes), then the child's work in treatment sessions may increase.

Idioms: Sayings, proverbs, and so forth; a type of figurative language; expressions that are peculiar to a language that cannot be understood by just understanding the meaning of individual words (e.g., *he kicked the bucket*).

Imitation: The child's response that immediately follows and reproduces a clinician's model; useful in teaching new skills; often a starting point in language treatment; the treatment protocols begin with clinician's modeling and the child's imitation; when the child correctly imitates on 5 consecutive trials, the clinician may fade modeling to introduce evoked trials.

Incidental teaching: A specific technique of milieu teaching (naturalistic language teaching) that helps teach elaborated language productions to children who independently initiate a communicative interaction with an adult; typically, an adult waits until a child shows an interest in something or initiates a topic of conversation; the adult then prompts the child to give an elaborate verbal response (e.g., "what do you want?"); the clinician further prompts if necessary and praises the child for elaborate productions.

Inferential meaning: That which is not explicitly stated but can be deduced (presumed) from what is said; one might, for instance, infer that the woman is going to bed when she says, late in the night, "I am tired"; generally difficult for children with language disorders; an advanced language treatment target.

Inflectional bound morphemes: Elements of language that are attached to a root word to add to the meaning of the root word, but not to create a new word; the regular plural s, for instance, an inflectional morpheme that is attached to nouns; good language treatment targets for children with language disorders.

Informative feedback: Increasing behaviors by providing feedback on the progress a child is making in learning a skill; an excellent form of verbal social reinforcement; the clinician might say, "Last time, you said 5 out of 10 sentences correctly; but today, you said 9 out of 10 sentences correctly!"

Intermittent schedule of reinforcement: Various ways of reinforcing only some of the correct responses while others go unreinforced; effective in strengthening newly learned skills; clinician typically reinforces all responses to begin with and thins out reinforcement by offering it for only some responses.

Joint attention: Two persons simultaneously paying attention to the same object or event; often refers to the behavior of a caregiver and child; necessary to teach various language skills.

Language: In the linguistic viewpoint, an arbitrary system of codes and symbols used to express ideas. In the behavioral viewpoint, measurable verbal behavior.

Language differences: Variations mostly in language production (and to some extent in comprehension) that may be associated with a particular linguistic or cultural community; must be taken into consideration in diagnosing a language disorder or prescribing treatment; language differences are not language disorders (e.g., lack of eye contact during conversation that is typical of a child's cultural background).

Language disorders: Lack of acceptable or effective social repertoire to affect the behaviors of other persons in social, educational, and occupational milieu or to be affected by the verbal behaviors of other persons; limited amount and quality of language productions; grammatical deficiencies; deficiencies in social communication; difficulty in meeting academic demands.

Language production: Speaking or communicating nonverbally; often contrasted with *comprehension.*

Language sample: Recording of a child's conversational or naturalistic verbal interaction with the clinician, a family member, or both; often necessary to diagnose a language disorder in a child; to be followed by baserates of selected language skills to be targeted for treatment.

Lexicon: The number of words a child produces and understands; synonymous with vocabulary.

Linguistics: An academic discipline concerned with the study of language.

Literacy skills: Reading and writing skills.

Maintenance: The continued production of clinically established skills over time and across situations; to have the child maintain clinically established skills, the clinician needs to train the family members, teachers, and others to evoke, prompt, and reinforce those skills in natural settings.

Maintenance strategies: Techniques that help extend treatment to natural settings; parent training and self-control strategies are the most effective.

Mand: A group of verbal responses that have motivational states as causes and often specify their own reinforcers; all requests, most questions, commands, and demands fall into this behavioral response class; a useful clinical target for children with language disorders.

Mand model: A milieu teaching method to establish joint attention as a cue for verbalization; when the child desires something, the clinician may model a request the child imitates and then gets what is requested.

Manual guidance: Providing physical assistance to prompt or execute a nonverbal response such as pointing to a picture; the clinician may ask "show me the car" (among several stimuli) and take the child's hand to point to the picture of a car.

Mean length of utterance: Calculated by counting the total number of morphemes and dividing that number by the total number of utterances in a language sample; a general measure of language development.

Metaphor: A saying that makes a comparison between two or more objects that are unlike each other (e.g., "The moon was a ghostly galleon . . ."); an abstract language target for children with language disorders who have mastered morphologic features and varied sentence structures.

Milieu teaching: A naturalistic treatment method in which the clinician reinforces child-initiated communicative interactions in response to environmental stimuli; includes *mand-model, delay,* and *incidental teaching.*

Model: The production of the target behavior by anyone who wants to teach a child an imitative response; effective in teaching a variety of skills to children; useful when a child will not produce a response without it; known to be an effective technique in teaching language skills to children.

Modeled trials: Baserate or treatment trials in which the clinician ask a question and immediately models the correct response for the child to imitate; when the child gives 5 consecutively correct, imitated responses, modeling is faded to introduce the evoked trials.

Morphemes: The smallest units of meaning within a language; all words are morphemes but not all morphemes (e.g., the plural *s* or the past tense *ed*) are words; good treatment targets for children with language disorders as they tend to omit them.

Morphologic skills: Production of words and words with suffixes and prefixes that help convey various forms of meaning; essential language skills; skills on which more complex language skills are built.

Morphology: The study of word structures, including whole words and bound morphemes (suffixes and prefixes).

Narrative skills: Telling stories or personal experiences with sufficient details, temporal sequence, characterization, and so forth; a pragmatic language skill; often deficient in children with language disorders; a good treatment target for children who have mastered the basic language skills (including the grammatic morphemes).

Negation: Forms of expressions or response classes that deny or negate assertions others make; expressions typically include such words as *no, not, cannot, did not,* and so forth.

Nonverbal communication: Communication without vocal productions; production of such nonvocal behaviors as signs, gestures, and nonvocal symbols to affect other people; a treatment target for children and adults who have extremely limited capacity for verbal productions.

Nonverbal prompts: Various signals or gestures the clinician gives to evoke the correct production of a target behavior; the clinician, for example, may manually demonstrate the motion of legs to suggest *walking*; the child may then say the word.

Obligatory contexts: Linguistic context in which a grammatic feature is required by the rules of grammar; for instance, the regular plural *s* is required when a speaker talks about plural objects (e.g., *two* books); useful in assessing or baserating the production of many grammatic morphemes.

Operational definition: A definition that describes that what is being defined in observable and measurable terms; most treatment targets are defined operationally (e.g., *the production of the plural morpheme in words at 90% accuracy*).

Partial model: A modeled stimulus that provides only a portion of the correct response; just enough for the child to imitate the response; a method to fade the influence of the full model; useful in promoting more spontaneous or naturalistic response.

Passive sentences: A sentence type in which the grammatical subject is the object of action; an indirect and longer way of expressing sentences (e.g., *the child was brought to the clinic by the mother*) in the active voice (e.g., *the mother brought the child to the clinic*).

Personal narratives: Talking about personal experiences; a useful advanced language treatment target for children with language disorders.

Pervasive developmental disorders (PDDs): Serious and multiple impairments in child development typically diagnosed in young children, usually before the age of 3; includes autism and Asperger's syndrome; many with PDDs need significant language treatment effort.

Picture Exchange Communication System (PECS): An augmentative and alternative communication training program in which the child is taught to exchange picture cards for desired items; shown to be effective in teaching children with language disorders, especially those with autism.

Pragmatics: The study of language production in social contexts; the study of social communication.

Primary language: The first language a child learns.

Primary reinforcement: A method of increasing target skills by providing consequences that promote the biological survival of a species; includes food items; not used in language treatment unless one is training mands for food and drinks; may be needed in teaching children who are profoundly retarded or have extremely limited verbal skills; the same as *unconditioned reinforcement.*

Probe: An assessment of generalized productions of clinically established skills; a final test of success of treatment; only untrained stimuli are presented during probes; no reinforcement or corrective feedback is offered on probe trials or assessment; the protocols include probes for most target behaviors.

Probe criterion: Generally, 90% correct responses given to untrained stimuli; if the child can produce the target skills in the context of new stimuli (typically encountered in natural settings), the teaching may be considered successful; protocols suggest that the clinician continue to teach new exemplars of a target skill until the probe criterion is met.

Prompt: A hint; may be verbal (e.g., vocal emphasis specified in the protocols) or nonverbal (e.g., a hand gesture); another special stimulus that is added or layered over another evoking or modeling stimuli; less than a full model; useful in fading modeling; known to be effective in teaching skills.

Protocols: Detailed and scripted plans for treatment, including baserates; as written in this book, protocols specify the roles the clinician and the client play in treatment sessions; the clinician and the child may follow the script to accomplish the treatment objectives.

Receptive language: Understanding spoken language; always inferred from a correct verbal response (e.g., correct answer to a question) or a nonverbal response (e.g., correctly pointing a named picture); separate training for comprehension may not be necessary in most cases; production training may be sufficient to induce both production and comprehension.

Reinforcers: Consequences provided contingent on a correct response that consists of verbal praise, objects, or opportunities for certain favorite activities; to be delivered immediately after a response is made; should increase the correct response rate to be called a reinforcer; the most powerful treatment technique.

Replicated: Treatment research that is repeated by either the same researcher or other researchers; helps demonstrate that the results of the original treatment research were reliable.

Response cost: Each incorrect response results in the loss of a reinforcer; a response reduction strategy; the clinician may withdraw a token for every incorrect response (when the child gets a token for every correct response).

Scripts: Describing a routine series of events or any series of events; description of procedures one can follow; treatment protocols illustrate scripts the clinicians follow in teaching a variety of skills to children with language disorders.

Secondary language: Language learned after learning the first or primary language; basis of bilingualism.

Secondary reinforcement: The use of social consequences to increase skills; verbal praise, included in almost all protocols, is a form of secondary reinforcement; based on past learning (unlike primary reinforcement).

Self-monitoring: A teachable skill that includes self-evaluation and self-correction (e.g., learning to stop as soon as an error is made); useful in response maintenance.

Setting generalization: Production of clinically established responses in such nonclinical settings as home, school, and social situations; a goal of all treatment.

Shaping: A treatment procedure designed to teach more complex skills by building upon a series of simple skills; the same as successive approximation; teaching a child to first say *walk* and then adding the present progressive *ing* to the verb is an example of shaping; useful and effective in language treatment.

Similes: Makes a comparison between two or more objects that are unlike each other and includes either the word *as* or *like* (e.g., "My love is like a red, red rose"); an advanced language treatment target for older children who have mastered the basic skills including the grammatic morphemes.

Social communication: More complex language skills exhibited in social contexts; includes the essential morphologic skills but goes beyond them; characterized by such complex skills as requests, questions, negation, passive sentences, idioms, expression of feelings and emotions; included in the second volume.

Specific language impairment: In the classical view, a language problem in a child who does not have any other clinical condition that would explain it or would be associated with it; according to a more recent view, a predominant language disorder but children may have subtle cognitive and sensory problems.

Speech: The production of sounds of a language; essential basic skill to produce language.

Spontaneous conversation: Discourse evoked by social and natural contexts and stimuli; an eventual goal of language treatment; the reason why special stimuli used in treatment (e.g., modeling and pictures) are faded.

Stimulus generalization: The production of already learned responses in relation to novel but similar stimuli; target of probes.

Synonyms: Different words that convey the same meaning; deficient in children with language disorders; a treatment target for children who have mastered the basic language skills.

Syntactic structures. Sentence structures and varied forms of sentences; deficient in children with language disorders; clinical treatment targets (e.g., *questions* and *passive sentences*).

Syntax: A collection of rules about word combinations and sentence structures within a language.

Systematic replication: Treatment research in which previous studies are repeated in different settings, by different researchers, using different clients to show that the technique will yield similar results under varied conditions and with different clinicians; techniques that are systematically replicated may be recommended for general practice; most techniques included in the protocols have been systematically replicated.

Tactile prompts: A special variety of nonverbal prompts involving touch known to be effective with some children, especially those with autism or developmental disability.

Target behavior: Any verbal or nonverbal skill a clinician wishes to teach a child; a larger class (e.g., *the production of the regular plural*) than a target response (e.g., the production of a particular exemplar such as *two books*).

Telegraphic speech: A type of condensed speech in which only essential words are used; typically missing are the grammatic morphemes; a characteristic of language disorders.

Textual prompts: Printed cues (e.g., a printed word) that help evoke a target response.

Time-out: A period of nonreinforcement, imposed response contingently, resulting in the reduction of that response; a method to reduce unwanted behaviors; the clinician may "freeze" for a few seconds as soon as the child makes an error and avoid eye contact; the child is asked not to talk during the duration of the time-out.

Topic initiation: The pragmatic language skill of introducing new topics for conversation; often deficient in children with language disorders; a useful clinical treatment target.

Topic maintenance: Continuous conversation on the same topic without abrupt introduction of new topics; a pragmatic language skill; deficient in children with language disorders; a useful clinical treatment target.

Unconditioned reinforcement: A method of increasing target skills by arranging consequences that have biological value to the recipients, synonymous with primary reinforcement; food and drink are examples; useful in case of severely impaired or nearly nonverbal children as well as in teaching mands of food and drink in any child.

Unreplicated: An unreplicated study is the first or the original study on a given procedure or concept; the study needs to be replicated before the results are known to be reliable or not.

Untrained stimuli (probe stimuli): Novel stimuli, not used in teaching a target skill but can evoke the same target skill; correct responses to untrained stimuli indicate generalized production; it means the teaching has been successful.

Verbal behavior: Behavior reinforced through the mediation of other persons; preferred to the term *language* in the behavioral viewpoint.

Verbal prompt: A special verbal stimulus designed to evoke a correct response; examples include "What do you say when you see two books?" or simply, "You say . . . "

References

American Speech-Language-Hearing Association. (2005). Child language disorders. Retrieved July 24, 2005 from www.asha.org/members/research/NOMS2/child_language.htm

Berko, J. (2001). *The development of language.* Boston, MA: Allyn and Bacon.

Bricker, D. (1993). Then, now, and the path between. In A. P. Kaiser & D. B. Gray (Eds.), *Enhancing children's communication: Research foundations for intervention* (pp. 11–31). Baltimore: Paul H. Brooks.

Brown, R. (1973). *A first language: The early stages.* Cambridge. MA: Harvard University Press.

Carr, C. and Associates. (Eds.). (1995). *Communication-based intervention for problem behavior.* Baltimore, MD: Paul H. Brookes.

Gleason, J. B. (2001). *The development of language* (5th ed.). Boston: Allyn & Bacon.

Goldstein, H. (2002). Communicative intervention for children with autism: A review of treatment efficacy. *Journal of Autism and Developmental Disabilities, 32*(5), 373–396.

Goldstein, H., & Hockenberger, E. H. (1991). Significant progress in child language intervention: An 11-year retrospective. *Research in Developmental Disabilities, 12,* 401–424.

Guess, D. (1969). A functional analysis of receptive language and productive speech: Acquisition of the plural morpheme. *Journal of Applied Behavior Analysis, 2,* 55–64.

Guess, D., & Baer, D. M. (1973). Some experimental analyses of linguistic development in institutionalized retarded children. In B. B. Lahey (Ed.), *The modification of language behavior* (pp. 3–60). Springfield, IL: Charles C. Thomas.

Guess, D., Sailor, W., Rutherford, G., & Baer, D. M. (1968). An experimental analysis of linguistic development: The productive use of the plural morpheme. *Journal of Applied Behavior Analysis, 1,* 225–235.

Hargis, C. H. (1977). *English syntax.* Springfield, IL: Charles C. Thomas.

Hart, B. (1985). Naturalistic language training techniques. In S. F. Warren & A. K. Rogers-Warren (Eds.), *Teaching functional language: Generalization and maintenance of language skills* (pp. 63–88). Austin, TX: Pro-Ed.

Hegde, M. N. (1980). An experimental-clinical analysis of grammatical and behavioral distinction between verbal auxiliary and copula. *Journal of Speech and Hearing Research, 23,* 864–877.

Hegde, M. N. (1998). *Treatment procedures in communicative disorders* (3rd ed.). Austin, TX: Pro-Ed.

Hegde, M. N., & Gierut, J. (1979). The operant training and generalization of pronouns and a verb form in language delayed children. *Journal of Communication Disorders, 12,* 23–34.

Hegde, M. N., & Maul, C. (2006). *Language disorders in children: An evidence-based approach to assessment and treatment.* Boston, MA: Allyn & Bacon.

Hegde, M. N., & McConn, J. (1981). Language training: Some data on response classes and generalization to an occupational setting. *Journal of Speech and Hearing Disorders, 46,* 353–358.

Hegde, M. N., Noll, M. J., & Pecora, R. (1979). A study of some factors affecting generalization of language training. *Journal of Speech and Hearing Disorders, 44,* 301–320.

Hulit, H., & Howard, M. R. (2002). *Born to talk.* Boston: Allyn and Bacon.

Kaiser, A. P., & Gray, D. P. (Eds.). (1993). *Enhancing children's communication: Research foundations for intervention.* Baltimore, MD: Paul H. Brookes.

Koegel, L. K., Koegel, R. L., & Dunlap, G. (Eds.). (1996). *Positive behavior support: Including people with difficult behavior in the community.* Baltimore, MD: Paul H. Brookes.

Maurice, C. (Ed.). (1996). *Behavioral intervention for young children with autism.* Austin, TX: Pro-Ed.

McLaughlin, S. (1998). *Introduction to language development.* Albany, NY: Delmar Thomson.

Reichle, J., & Wacker, D. P. (Eds.). (1993). *Communicative alternatives to challenging behavior: Integrating functional assessment and intervention strategies.* Baltimore, MD: Paul H. Brookes.

Risley, T. R., & Reynolds, N. J. (1970). Emphasis as a prompt for verbal imitation. *Journal of Applied Behavior Analysis, 3,* 185–190.

Schumaker, J., & Sherman, J. A. (1970). Training generative verb usage by imitation and reinforcement procedures. *Journal of Applied Behavior Analysis, 3,* 273–287.

Streng, A. H. (1972). *Syntax, speech & hearing.* New York: Grune & Stratton.

Warren, S. F. (1992). Facilitating basic vocabulary acquisition with milieu teaching procedures. *Journal of Early Intervention, 16,* 235–251.

Warren, S. F., & Kaiser, A. P. (1986). Incidental language teaching: A critical review. *Journal of Speech and Hearing Disorders, 51,* 291–299.

Warren, S. F., & Rogers-Warren, A. K. (1985). Teaching functional language. In S. F. Warren & A. K. Rogers-Warren (Eds.), *Teaching functional language* (pp. 3–23). Austin, TX: Pro-Ed.

Appendix A

First Few Functional Words

First Few Functional Words

Clothing									
belt	bib	boots	hat	jacket	shirt	shoes	socks	sweater	pants
skirt	blouse	nightie	pajama	towel	sheet	rag			

Food									
apple	banana	bread	cake	candy	cheese	chips	cookie	crackers	egg
gum	burger	juice	meat	melon	milk	orange	peach	pickle	pizza
soda	soup	spaghetti	taco	toast	water				

ball	bike	blocks	doll	swing	tricycle	car	train	truck	plane	puzzle
Barbie	skateboard	teddy bear							

Furniture and Household Items									
bed	blanket	clock	crib	door	drawer	light	pillow	telephone	sofa
chair	table	spoon	plate	pot	cup	fork	mug	knife	scissors
towel									

Kinship Terms								
mother	father	brother	sister	son	daughter	grandfather	grandmother	parent
uncle	aunt	cousin						

Adjectives									
big	little	large	small	tall	short	long	high	low	happy
sad	red	blue	yellow	green	purple	pink	orange		

Animals									
dog	kitty	fish	bird	bat	horse	cow	chicken	zebra	pony
elephant	tiger	lion	snake	hippo	rhino	bear	monkey	rabbit	gerbil

Appendix B

Baserate Recording Sheet

Baserate Recording Sheet

[Type Your Clinic's Name Here]		
Name:	Date:	File #:
DOB/Age:	Clinician:	
Disorder:	Target Behavior:	

Goal: [type-in]	Trials	
Target Responses	**Evoked**	**Modeled**
1.		
2.		
3.		
4.		
5.		
6.		
7.		
8.		
9.		
10.		
11.		
12.		
13.		
14.		
15.		
16.		
17.		
18.		
19.		
20.		
Percent correct baserate		

Note: + = Correct response; – = Incorrect response; 0 = no response.

Appendix C

Treatment Recording Sheet

Treatment Recording Sheet

[Type Your Clinic's Name Here]		
Name:	Date:	File #:
DOB/Age:	Clinician:	
Disorder:	Target Behavior:	
Goal: [type-in]		

Clinician's Comments:

Scoring: Correct: ✓   Incorrect or no response: X

Target skills	Discrete Trials														
	1	2	3	4	5	6	7	8	9	10	11	12	13	14	15
1.															
2.															
3.															
4.															
5.															
6.															
7.															
8.															
9.															
10.															

Appendix D

Probe Recording Sheet

Probe Recording Sheet

[Type Your Clinic's Name Here]			
Name:	Date:		File #:
Age:	Clinician:		
Disorder:	Target Behavior:		
Name:	Date:	Session #:	
Age:	Clinician:		
Disorder: Language	Target:	(Probe)	
Untrained Stimuli (UT)	**Score: + correct; - incorrect or no responses**		
1.		(UT)	
2.		(UT)	
3.		(UT)	
4.		(UT)	
5.		(UT)	
6.		(UT)	
7.		(UT)	
8.		(UT)	
9.		(UT)	
10.		(UT)	
Percent correct probe (Criterion: 90%)			

Index